DR SEBI BIBLE

To Complete Guide to Everything You Need to Know About Dr. Sebi's Treatments and Cures for Any Disease, Alkaline Diet and Encyclopedia of Herbs.

By Kelly Outtara

Table of Contents

Introduction

It is true that health is wealth; however, many disregards the call to give their health the attention it deserves for a variety of reasons. And the main reason is insufficient time, but when we get sick, we have no choice but to pause that same time and all our activities.

Often, people fail to realize that diseases and illnesses do not just emerge from nowhere but accumulate over time. Your body must have been sending you signs and signals, but you ignored all of them as you continued on your way.

Your body is alarming you: when you feel tired quickly, experience digestive distress, become allergic to food, start feeling unhealthy even though you eat well, feel weak in your joints, are not as mentally sharp as you were, feel stressed out quickly, etc.

Having said that, we can compare this to the way a car always gives off signals before it breaks down, such as starting after several attempts, jerking, or making some strange sounds when it does so. So, if you are experiencing all the above-stated symptoms, it indicates that your immune system has been reacting to an anomaly or an impending danger posed by pathogens. Therefore, when we receive these signals, we must take immediate action to ensure the return of our body system to usual.

In most cases, the best thing to do is to detox, which entails the removal of unwanted material from our bodies. Although you may have heard of detox before, you may not be familiar in details with the concept. Nevertheless, you need not worry, as it is thoroughly explained in this book.

There are many people who are apprehensive about the idea of detox. It may seem daunting or too demanding to them. Hence, this book explains a number of natural ways and steps you can follow to detox your body from contaminants. This book is a collection of all the guidelines by Dr. Sebi, a renowned herbalist healer who places a greater emphasis on healthy eating habits that one needs to adopt to detoxify their body.

In order to take full advantage of Dr. Sebi's alkaline diet, this book offers a three-step process to help you detox your body naturally and safely. First of all, we need to get you to understand what Dr. Sebi's diet is all about because we cannot walk around blindfolded in ignorance and expect to get something good out of it. Therefore, before you take any further action, you must have a clear and thorough understanding of the diet that you intend to follow.

When you have a thorough understanding of a diet, you are then ready for the second step, which is to discover the ingredients and items it involves. Knowing the principles underlying how a car works do not mean you also know how it works at all, so you need to understand all of the different components of the car in order to know how it works effectively. The best drivers know not only how to drive their cars but also every part of them.

A similar idea applies to Dr. Sebi's diet, where you need to learn not only how the diet works but also what foods are allowed and what foods are prohibited, as this will give you some insight into how to plan your meals. In step 3, you will need to plan out your weekly meals. Although a guide to the 7-day meal plan has already been provided, you can plan your own course from the list of approved foods in step 2. This three-step plan will help you unlock your body's natural detoxification.

Who is Dr. Sebi?

Dr. Sebi, otherwise known as Alfred Darrington Bowman, was born in Spanish Honduras, more specifically in the village of Ilanga. The date of Alfred Darrington Bowman's birth was November 26, 1933, and he passed away on August 6, 2016. Although he lived in Honduras throughout his life, he never identified himself as an African Honduran, only as an African living there. It is believed that he had two marriages and survived by 17 children in his lifetime.

His reputation as a healer and herbalist was widely praised. He was a self-educated herbalist and healer who practiced extensively in the US during the latter part of his life. Additionally, he was a biochemist, naturalist, and pathologist. A special and unique method of healing created by Dr. Sebi centered around rooted herbs was unique and developed by him. During his career, he carefully studied the herbs found in rivers and forests of Africa, in South and Central and Northern America, the Caribbean, and some other regions.

Dr. Sebi was diagnosed with diabetes, obesity, impotence, and asthma when he first came to the United States of America. It was only after orthodox doctors had treated him to no avail with modern drugs and traditional Western medicine that he was referred to a Mexican herbalist who would be able to help him. This Mexican herbalist's success in healing all the conditions he suffered from, as well as the knowledge he gained studying under his grandmother, 'mama hay,' led him to develop a natural plant cell food compound.

Notably, he developed an unorthodox method of creating these compounds, which was possible after years of acquiring empirical knowledge that enabled him to develop this method. His compounds' sole purpose is to clean and revitalize all the cells within the body. Despite opposition and objections, he devoted 30 years of his life to this cause until his death.

Dr. Sebi's approach to diseases was influenced by the famous African methodology of medicine, which is mainly based on herbal remedies (botanicals). By using these remedies, the body can be cleansed of toxins by a process known as detoxification. Through this method, the body is restored to an alkaline state, which means that it is no longer allowed to grow and develop pathologies and diseases in an acidic state.

A natural vegetable cell food compound is at the center of this remedy. Dr. Sebi believed that because of the components of this compound, it was capable of revitalizing damaged tissues in a body that has been weakened by acidity. In order to accomplish this goal, we need to replenish the minerals in our bodies and get rid of the accumulated toxins.

Such toxins primarily affect the kidneys, lymph glands, liver, and skin. As a result, Dr. Sebi devised a nutritional plan based on an alkaline state of body balance. It does not merely address the pathology or disease but emphasizes the patient's entire well-being to boost their recovery. There's no doubt that cell foods play a huge role in creating an environment that is conducive to good health and healing.

Dr. Sebi's life work aimed to advocate for the benefits of alkalizing the body through one's diet (food intake). Specifically, he claims that dead food prevents the body from performing the natural process of cleansing itself, which is necessary in order to maintain good health. Foods that fall under this category include sugar, processed foods, alcohol, meat, poultry, fried foods, etc.

According to him, if one eliminates the foods mentioned above from one's diet, the body would be able to cleanse naturally (detox), eventually allowing one's body to function properly, thus leading to a healthy body and life. Foods considered to be alkaline in nature include raw nuts, vegetables containing no starch, naturally ripened fruits, and grains (such as kamut, rye, and quinoa). He continued to claim that with the help of this simple procedure, he was able to cure chronic illnesses such as diabetes, cancer, AIDS, blindness, etc.

Throughout his professional career, Dr. Sebi has consistently shared his deep-rooted knowledge of traditional herbs and their constituents in his office in Brooklyn, New York, and Dr. Sebi's LLC, located in La Ceiba, Honduras. According to Dr. Sebi, he believes herbs and a strict vegan diet can treat all ailments, as well as AIDS, which he denies is the result of HIV infection.

A closer look at these claims allows one to label them pseudoscientific. Dr. Sebi has created and developed various products, including Horadin, Cell Proliferate Eva-Therapeutic Salve, Nervino, Hair Food, Limphaslin, Uturin, Testee II, and others. He claims to have an all-inclusive package that costs 1,500 dollars that is supposed to detoxify the body cells by breaking down acids, mucus, and toxins for easy removal from the body.

Even though Alfred Bowman did not have formal training in medicine, he used the title and name, Dr. Sebi. It's why some attorneys, doctors with licenses, and other protection agencies call him a quack in the US. He was regarded as a threat by many multinational medical companies.

He got arrested several times for practicing without a license. The attorney general of New York, Robert Adams, charged Dr. Sebi and sent him to court in 1987. His indictment resulted from two counts of illegal practice of medicine without a license, fraudulent claims of therapeutic abilities of his products and services, including a claim that he had cured some diseases, including AIDS, with the help of his products and services. The Food and Drug Administration also accused him of illegally selling unapproved products.

These charges were brought against him when he placed advertisements in the Amsterdam News and Village Voice papers claiming that he had the ability to cure diseases like sickle cell anemia, AIDS, herpes, and more. He refused to take down the advertisement before the lawsuits despite having been instructed by the New York Department of Consumer Affairs and the Attorney General.

As an initial fee, 500 dollars was required of his clients, and later appointments were about 80 dollars. In the advertisement, he said that USHA had already cured AIDS. When the judge heard the case, he demanded a patient who could attest he had cured him. Eventually, he was released after bringing over 70 patients.

After the Brooklyn supreme court's verdict, Dr. Sebi gained great fame. It was reported by Amsterdam news that the prosecutor recovered tapes from two undercover agents who infiltrated Dr. Sebi's institute. The purpose of this was to catch him making medical diagnoses.

Even though the prosecutor had provided the jury with a copy of these recordings, they were not convinced that Dr. Sebi had indeed made the diagnosis of medical malpractice. This verdict was very important because it ushered in the global recognition of the African biomineral balance (a therapeutic method developed by USHA that is suited for the nutritional requirements of Africans based on their genetic structure), as claimed by Simeon Greenaway, the attorney for Dr. Sebi. In his many interviews, Dr. Sebi often refers to this victory as one of his greatest achievements.

In an interview five years ago, Dr. Sebi claimed that he had defended himself when he appeared on the Rock Newman program. "The judge instructed me to provide one patient to support my claim, and I provided over 70." Additionally, he stated that when his mother first heard that he had cured over ten HIV patients, she was very concerned and worried the authorities would investigate.

The interviewee asked Dr. Sebi about the process he used to cure a patient with AIDS. He explained to the interviewer that he only gave the patient a compound that helped clean his cells and restructured his diet. Additionally, he removed from his diet foods containing lactose, carbonic acid, starch, milk, meat, and uric acid. He said that the patient started to notice improvements within 24 hours of doing this.

However, before his interview, successful legal proceedings were brought against USHA. The court, in this instance, ruled that Dr. Sebi's statements were baseless. As a result, Dr. Sebi's firm was obliged to sign an agreement prohibiting him from making claims about their medicines' medicinal qualities. The agreement prohibited USHA, Fig Tree Institute, and their directors, officers, agents, employees, successors, Dr. Sebi, and Mama Bowman from making any claims, whether written or oral, that their products or services could cure or relieve or even change the course or direction of any disease or physical condition such as sickle cell anemia, AIDS, pains, leukemia, lupus, injuries, herpes, deformities, ulcers, and so on.

He was fined 900 dollars in addition to additional limitations. Following the lawsuit, Dr. Sebi traveled to California and relocated his USHA research centers. In California, he built and enlarged his profession. Top celebrities such as Michael Jackson, Lisa Lopes, John Travolta, Steven Seagal, and Eddie Murphy were among his clients.

Dr. Sebi said Michael Jackson was his patient in 2004 before the singer was accused of child abuse. He also stated that while working with him in Colorado, he helped the celebrity overcome his painkiller addiction (Morphine and Demerol) by using his dietary treatment (African Bio-Electric Cell Food).

Dr. Sebi then sued Michael Jackson, claiming that Jackson's brother did not completely compensate him when he gave him $10,000. He claimed he was due 380,000 dollars and wanted an extra 600,000 in damages for the time he spent making court appointments, forcing him to postpone visits with other customers and other events.

This prompted Jackson's publicist to publish a statement rejecting Dr. Sebi's allegations, claiming that his client did not have a painkiller addiction and did not undergo any professional therapy from the self-proclaimed doctor. The judge dropped the case in 2015 owing to a lack of prosecution.

Dr. Sebi was detained on May 28 at the Juan Manuel Galvez international airport in Honduras with 37,000 USD in his possession. Although he was freed until his court appearance, he was detained again on June 3 of that year by Honduras' counterpart to the FBI, the Ministerio Publico, and accused of money laundering.

Official documents of his arrest have yet to be revealed in order to clarify the grounds for his detention, since having that amount of money in his possession would not have been unusual for a man like himself with top celebrities as clientele. Dr. Sebi was detained for almost a month while awaiting trial. His relatives attempted but failed to secure his release. He was later transported to the hospital on August 6 due to pneumonia. He died on the way to the hospital, unfortunately, at the age of 82.

Major news outlets did not cover Dr. Sebi's life, works/claims, or death. This is part of the fuel for the conspiracy theory alleging multibillion-dollar pharmaceutical firms were against the self-made doctor and people knowing about him, his diet, his goods, and his death.

According to the conspiracy theorist, a guy who claimed to have cured AIDS and supported his claims in court by offering victims he had healed would make headlines in every news agency. They claim that his non-viral public appearance was manipulated by pharmaceutical firms because "there is no profit in a cure. " They believe that the pharmaceutical industry needs people to be sick to generate money, and they don't receive anything if they are well."

And Dr. Sebi was not only selling wellness, but he was doing it without synthetic pharmaceuticals, simply encouraging and directing people towards a healthy lifestyle through proper nutrition and, in certain circumstances, the use of pure herbal remedies. This would discourage individuals from using pharmaceuticals, putting a dent in the purses of big pharmaceutical giants.

This conspiracy idea also links to the death of Nipsey Hussle, a Los Angeles-based rapper. Before his untimely death, the rapper said in a breakfast club interview in 2018 that he was working on a documentary on Dr. Sebi's 1985 trial against New York when he claimed to have cured AIDS.

He believed the tale was essential and that people would want to know more about someone who not only claimed but also supported the cure for AIDS. He claimed to have joked that the endeavor may lead to his death. These theories argued that the rapper's death resulted from pharmaceutical firms attempting to keep Dr. Sebi's work from becoming public.

BOOK 1
What is Dr. Sebi's Diet?

Dr. Sebi's diet consists of an alkaline-centered diet and herbal supplements. Dr. Sebi thinks that diseases and illnesses are the result of acid and mucus buildup in the body. Disease and sickness, on the other hand, cannot exist in an alkaline environment. As a result, his diet serves to detoxify or cleanse the body and restore its alkaline balance.

However, there is no scientific evidence to support this assertion. The diet is plant-based, and it forbids the eating of all animal products such as milk, meat, and so on. It is quite close to a vegan diet, but it does not allow the intake of all plants, particularly those that are acidic.

Dr. Sebi's diet forbids seedless fruits and allows only naturally cultivated cereals. This diet also forbids the eating of any artificial and hybrid foods. The herbalist thinks that following this diet strictly would not only heal you of ailments, but will also help your body become immune to them by establishing an alkaline environment in the body that inhibits disease growth and development.

What is Alkaline food?

The body's pH, temperature, hydration, nutrition availability, and other elements are all crucial for the normal functioning of its cells and tissues. Depending on how it is measured, pH can be acidic or alkaline. It features a scale that ranges from 0 to 14. When the pH falls below 7 (from 6 to 0), it is considered to be acidic. When it is 7, it is neutral, and when it is greater than 7 (between 8 and 14), it is alkalizing.

However, the body normally works slightly over neutral, at 7.365. The pH of the blood is the most vital and well-protected in the body, since any minor change in its pH can be devastating. When the blood pH level falls below 6, the person has already entered a coma. A simple test, which may easily be done at home, should be performed to identify whether the body is acidic or alkaline. To begin, obtain a test strip and dip it in either saliva or urine. Then wait and see the colour that appears. The test strip has a colour code.

While the liver is in charge of detoxifying the body (including the blood), the kidney is the primary organ in charge of maintaining the blood's alkaline pH level. The kidney guarantees that the body can perform its functions as a conduit for both oxygen and other essential substances.

The kidney does this by filtering excessively acidic components in the blood and excreting them through urine. The body then uses its alkaline reserve to naturally adjust the pH level.

However, by constantly consuming acidic meals, which eventually deposit acid in our system, we overwork our kidney by putting it to tax digesting and excreting excess acids. After a while, our kidney becomes overworked and can no longer keep up with the amount of excess acid, resulting in acid accumulation in the tissues and subsequent disease development and deterioration of our health.

This is because it inhibits the body's ability to cleanse and heal itself, making the body more susceptible to illness. Studies have revealed that a 'acidic inner terrain' (a concentrated acidic environment, sometimes known as "acidosis") can cause muscle degeneration, kidney stones, decreased bone density, diabetes, arthritis, cancer, and other health problems. Other indications of acidosis are listed below:

- Low energy which will lead to weakness
- Chronic fatigue
- Shortage of breath
- Digestive disorder
- Acne and headache
- Osteoporosis
- Weak immune system
- Candida and other infections
- Allergies
- Heart disorder
- Slow recovery time especially after exercise
- Brittle hair and nails, etc.

We've demonstrated that it's difficult for the body to constantly cleanse and neutralise acids before they build and become toxic to the cell by modifying the overall environment in the body. And pollutants from the foods we consume, the water we drink, nicotine, pharmaceuticals, and other sources have all contributed significantly to the high acidity level.

However, this increase in the acidity level of the body is caused not only by our food, but also by our body performing its daily duties. Acids are produced by the body through the processes of breathing, muscular contraction, and digestion (although from some specific kinds of food). Stress, lack of sleep, and a polluted environment can all contribute to the formation of acids in the body.

The acidic content of food does not immediately harm the body, but rather the accumulation of chemical waste deposits from food over time. Consumption of refined and processed foods, as well as any animal products, hastens the accumulation process. The reason for this is that when these items are introduced to our diet, they can create up to 100mEq of acid every day. This amount is about double what our bodies can normally manage.

So, while our bodies can manage their acidity levels, our food may either impede or aid the process. As a result, adding alkaline foods to our diet can help our system maintain the alkalinity of the body for optimum functioning and wellness. When the body is acidic, it requires the consumption of important minerals in order to neutralise the acid in the body. Some plant-based diets are alkaline, whereas animal products (meat, eggs, and so on) and processed meals are acidic.

The body's cells require an alkaline environment to operate optimally, protect against harmful microorganisms, and stop and repair cellular damage. The purpose of an alkaline diet is to adjust our bodies' pH through food. Because, as previously said, the food we eat after metabolism produces waste that might be alkaline or acidic. As a result, alkaline diets, such as Dr. Sebi's, are focused with managing the pH of metabolic waste from the food we eat by following a rigorous healthy plant-based diet plan.

An alkaline diet, also known as an alkaline acid diet, an alkaline ash diet, or an acid-alkaline diet, arose from an osteoporosis research theory known as the acid ash hypothesis. This concept was developed by Claude Bernard, a French scientist. He tested and observed that when he switched a rabbit's food from a carnivore diet (i.e. meat) to a herbivore diet (i.e. plant), the pH of its urine became more alkaline, as opposed to the prior diet's high acidic level.

He then went on to examine the acidity and chemical qualities of the remaining meals, which were combusted in a calorimeter for explosives, also known as "ash." He arrived to the conclusion that when meals are digested, they leave behind residues in the body that are akin to alkaline ash or acid ash, much as those combusted in the bomb calorimeter.

A nutritionist, including our own Dr. Sebi, refined this concept in the twentieth century. These nutritionists classified food particles into two types: anions (which are negatively charged) and cations (known as positive charge). When anion particles such as phosphate, sulphate, or chloride are broken down, they produce acid. After the metabolic response, meals containing cation particles such as calcium, potassium, or potassium become alkaline. This diet is often referred to as the alkaline electric diet.

How to Start Dr. Sebi Diet?

Dr. Sebi's alkaline diet focuses on lowering mucus and acid levels in the body by following a rigorous meal plan. Based on Dr. Sebi's 30 years of plant and herbal study, this guide contains a list of foods that are either restricted or authorised. This list includes all non-hybrid plants that produce alkali as well as certain herbal supplements to revitalise the cells.

Following this eating plan would require abstaining from dairy products, meat, sweets, and any processed foods. This would surely assist you in maintaining your weight. This diet might be used with fasting with the help of a doctor to achieve the desired results.

The first step of this diet is the most difficult since your body craves sweets. However, as you progress through the diet regimen, it improves. In addition, following this guidance would need you to begin preparing the majority of your meals at home because most restaurants do not provide a menu fit for this healthy lifestyle.

Dr. Sebi classified food into six types: raw, living, hybrid, dead, genetically modified (GMO), and pharmaceuticals. Foods that fit into the latter four categories must be avoided at all costs, including genetically engineered plants and hybrid plants. Foods to avoid include chicken, meat (while they come under the live and uncooked categories, they should be avoided), shellfish, sweets, alcohol, iodized salt, and many more. He urges people to eat foods that are raw or live, but they must be plant-based. Naturally ripe fruits, raw nuts, grains, non-starchy vegetables, rye, quinoa, leafy greens, and many more are examples of these foods. These dishes are also known as electrified foods.

This diet plan must be rigorously followed by adhering to the following rules: • Only foods included in Dr. Sebi's diet or nutritional guide may be ingested.

- A gallon (3.8 litres) of fresh spring water should be consumed everyday.

- Dr. Sebi's herbal supplements should not be used within an hour of taking any medicine.

- No hybrid foods or animal products are authorised.

- Alcohol should be avoided.

- Wheat is not permitted, and only naturally produced seeds indicated in the handbook should be used.

- Avoid using the microwave since it ruins your meals.

- All seedless fruits are prohibited, and tinned food is not authorised.

Anyone who wishes to follow this electric diet plan must acquire Dr. Sebi's herbal cell supplements in order to get the diet's full stated effects. Dr. Sebi's official website is where you may buy his products. The advance package (including 10 goods) costs 750 dollars, while the all-inclusive package (containing twenty things) costs 1,500 dollars. The all-inclusive bundle is intended for rapid cell cleansing and healing. It also provides settings dependent on the user's gender.

If you cannot afford any of the bundles, you can purchase individual things. Purchase products that are high in protein components. This is because the body cannot function without protein, and Dr. Sebi's diet prohibited the eating of high-protein foods such as beans, soy products, pork, lentils, and so on.

Aside from that, there is no special product advice; you might buy items containing the nutrients that you require at the moment and for your needs. Bio Ferro, for example, functions as a blood cleanser, improves liver function, boosts immunity, aids in weight loss, and generally improves overall body health.

BOOK 2
Benefits of Dr. Sebi Diet

So, what exactly is the benefit of this diet? And why is Dr. Sebi's diet healthy?

Dr. Sebi's diet urges individuals to consume more fruits and vegetables while consuming fewer processed meats and high-fat dairy items. Following this diet can assist persons with renal disease improve their health. As will be detailed further below, some of the benefits of an alkaline diet include: preventing the degradation of bone density and tissues caused by the availability of too much acid in the body, which can deprive us of key mineral minerals that an alkaline diet provides.

Provides protection for muscle mass and bone density

Researchers believe that consuming more alkalizing fruits and vegetables protects against Sarcopenia (decreased bone strength and muscle atrophy caused by ageing), and that the minerals provided by an alkaline diet play an important role in the formation and maintenance of bone structure.

An alkaline diet promotes bone health by balancing the ratio of key minerals such as calcium, magnesium, and phosphate required for sustaining lean muscle mass and bone formation. The alkaline diet also improves growth hormone synthesis and vitamin D absorption, which helps protect bones and reduces other chronic health issues.

Brings an increase in muscle mass

Even if it is far from your objective, having increased muscle mass allows you to do many things. A high degree of muscle mass aids in increasing your metabolic rate and burning fat. Dr. Sebi's diet is recognised for preserving and increasing muscle mass.

There is a research involving two groups of males. One group followed a healthy eating plan, whereas the other followed the 80/20 rule. Both groups followed the identical diet and exercise routine. The group that followed the 80/20 rule is of particular importance to us.

Over the course of eight weeks, both groups acquired the same amount of muscle mass, with the exception that the alkaline diet group shed more fat. It was clear that not only does the alkaline diet help you increase muscle mass, but it also helps you reduce fat. This is due to the enhanced growth hormone obtained as a result of alkalizing. This hormone causes less muscle breakdown and greater fat burn, which is why this diet is essential for maintaining and increasing muscle mass.

Boosts your energy level

Feeling weary and lethargic as a result of a sugar crash leads the insulin level to rise, lowering your energy level and sending a signal to your brain to rest. You have greater energy on an Alkaline diet since there are no insulin spikes during the day.

Because your body is in a typical starving phase, you have greater energy because it enters a fight or flight reaction. This is when your body releases adrenaline throughout the day, providing you with the energy you need to get by since your body believes it needs to go on a hunting journey to get food. It is important to note that you will feel less energy at the start of your diet journey since your body is still adjusting to these new adjustments. After the first week or two, you will notice that you have more energy to complete more work, which will make you feel a lot better.

Prevents strokes and hypertension

One of the anti-aging advantages of Dr. Sebi's alkaline diet is an increase in growth hormone synthesis and a decrease in inflammation, which has resulted in protection against common health concerns such as hypertension, stroke, high cholesterol, kidney stones, and enhanced cardiovascular health. According to research, growth hormone improves body composition and decreases the risk factors for heart disease, which is the leading cause of mortality in the United States.

Every year, an estimated 610,000 Americans die as a result of it. Another cause is an unhealthy lifestyle, which includes bad diet and a lack of physical activity. When you avoid red meat and eat a diet high in low-fat dairy, seeds, fruits, and vegetables, you lower your risk of heart disease. A healthy body weight results from consuming an alkaline diet, which creates less calories, which can also benefit your heart.

Helps in reducing chronic pain and inflammation in the body

With the help of research, we can identify a link between the alkaline diet and lower levels of chronic pain. Persistent acidosis has been linked to chronic back pain, muscular spasms, migraines, inflammation, joint pain, and menstruation symptoms. A study conducted in Germany by the Society for Minerals and Trace Elements discovered that 76 of 82 patients with chronic back pain who were given a daily dose of alkaline supplement for four weeks reported a significant reduction in pain as measured by the "Arhus rating scale for people with low back pain."

Cleanses and detoxifies your body

Detoxifying the body is essential for living a long and healthy life. There are several techniques available for people to detox their bodies, some of which do not generally work. The Alkaline diet has been shown time and again to help cleanse the human body on both a cellular and intestinal level, making it a great cleaning agent when it comes to the body.

On a cellular level, an alkaline diet detoxifies the body by eliminating unhealthy cells and replacing them with healthier, stronger cells through a process known as autophagy. This process has several advantages, including a better immune system, illness prevention, insulin sensitivity, and a lower chance of cancer, which is fantastic news.

When one considers how the body may be detoxified with the Alkaline diet on a digestive level, one can see that there is a link between the stomach and the brain. According to research, if the digestive system isn't operating properly, the brain won't be either, which is why the human stomach is referred to as a second brain.

It is critical for the gut to be clean and functioning correctly, and the Alkaline diet assists in this endeavour by clearing waste and garbage out of the intestines. Also, giving the digestive system a break by not eating for a period of time is one method of cleansing the stomach because eating all the time does not allow the body to clean itself.

When you begin fasting, your body will gradually begin to cleanse itself of any toxins existing in your stomach. This procedure improves your ability to think and digest meals. By detoxifying your body with an Alkaline diet, you minimise your risk of disease and increase your longevity.

Boosts vitamin absorption and prevents magnesium deficiency

Magnesium insufficiency has resulted in cardiac difficulties, migraines, sleep problems, anxiety, and muscular discomfort. Magnesium is required for the activation of vitamin D, which is essential for general immunological and endocrine function. Furthermore, magnesium is required for the proper functioning of hundreds of biological functions and enzyme systems.

Enhances immune function and protects against cancer

When cells lack adequate minerals to effectively oxygenate the body or dispose of waste, the entire body suffers. Our bodies accumulate infections and poisons, which weakens our immune system when vitamin absorption is hampered by mineral loss and can promote the formation of malignant cells.

Although whether Dr. Sebi's diet may prevent cancer or help with chemotherapy is still debatable and untested, a published study in the British Journal of Radiology discovered evidence that malignant cell death was more likely in an alkaline body rather than an acidic body.

An alkaline change in pH is thought to be connected with cancer prevention due to an adjustment in electric charges and the release of basic protein components. The alkaline diet has been demonstrated to be more advantageous for several chemotherapeutic medicines that require a higher pH to act properly, and alkalinity reduces the risk of cancer and inflammation.

Significant evidence from a 2010 study reveals that eating more vegetables and fruits and limiting meat consumption may help prevent cancer. The American Cancer Society (ACS) recommends a diet rich in fruits, vegetables, and whole grains as opposed to consuming processed meals, soft drinks, and various high-fat foods.

Enhances insulin sensitivity

It is well knowledge that an Alkaline diet improves insulin sensitivity. But how does insulin function in the body?

When you consume a meal, your body's insulin level rises and is utilised to transfer food to your fat reserves or muscle. When you have too much glycogen in your circulation, your body transfers it to your fat storage as energy, but if you are insulin sensitive, your muscle store receives the glycogen and utilises it for energy. When you are insulin sensitive, you are more likely to burn up all of the glycogen in your diet quickly without having to convert it to fat.

The Alkaline diet works to cure insulin resistance by depleting all glycogen reserves and forcing your body to utilise fat stores. Eating again would just lead the body to utilise up all of the glycogen and transfer it directly to the muscle mass to be used for energy rather than storing it as fat.

This is how the Alkaline diet makes you more insulin sensitive. Some of the advantages of being more insulin sensitive include having greater mental energy and less brain fog, having less fat stored in the body, which is perfect for losing weight or even gaining muscle because most of the energy is sent to muscle storage. Insulin sensitivity also aids in the treatment of type 2 diabetes. These advantages contribute to a healthy existence in general.

It helps in maintaining a healthy weight

Foods that generate an alkaline environment are also anti-inflammatory. Eating more of these items and reducing your intake of acid-forming meals makes it simpler to lose weight since the diet causes the body to attain normal leptin levels and inflammation, which influences your hunger and fat-burning skills.

Because the alkaline diet is minimal in calories, you feel quite pleased consuming the quantity of calories required by the body. While the Alkaline diet's focus is not on fat reduction, following the Alkaline diet's meal plan may surely assist defend against obesity. If weight loss is your ultimate objective, a keto alkaline diet that is low in carbohydrates is one of the finest options to attempt.

Sebi's diet keeps you away from diseases

We need to figure out how to lower the risk of illnesses for total health and well-being, and that is where the Alkaline diet comes in.

Alzheimer's and Parkinson's disease are two of the numerous ailments that Dr. Sebi's diet can help with. It has been demonstrated that food can help reduce the risk of neurologic illnesses and improve brain health. According to several research, Dr. Sebi's diet can help lower the likelihood of depression, and while most people do not consider this a disorder, the benefits cannot be understated.

According to a 2010 research on overweight women, the diet has been shown to lower LDL cholesterol levels and assist relieve health issues such as high blood pressure.

The Alkaline diet aids in the reduction of type 2 diabetes in people who suffer from it. Although it is not recommended, if you have type 2 diabetes, you can try this because a research on males found that the Alkaline diet helped them quit using insulin. This merely demonstrates how effective the diet is, with several extensive studies supporting its significance in decreasing the risk of diabetes and helping patients recover from a variety of conditions.

Those suffering from a disease or other ailment can have their immune system increased with the Alkaline diet, which helps them prevent minor illnesses such as the common flu. With these and many more rejuvenating characteristics of the Alkaline diet, one should weigh the benefits before contemplating the drawbacks.

It can improve your kidney health

According to a 2017 study, the usual diet in the United States has more acid, which can be harmful to the kidney. Kidney disease progresses slowly for people who have it, and symptoms improve when a reduced acid diet is taken. A person with renal illness has a more difficult time eliminating acid from the blood.

For patients with chronic kidney illness, there is no need to adopt a specialised alkaline diet; merely avoid acidic, rich diets and heavy alkaline foods. This is how the kidney maintains the pH of the blood. The abundance of organic salt found in vegetables and fruits helps lower acid loads in the body and is an excellent means of regulating your pH level.

Because the body is not yet sensitive to potassium, an alkaline diet rich in vegetables and fruits is especially beneficial during the early stages of renal disease. According to a new study, eating more fruits and vegetables is beneficial to the kidney since it helps the organs enhance their performance during sickness.

An increase in the production of neurotrophic growth factors

The alkaline diet has a wonderful impact on the brain which happens with the aid of BDNF- a brain-derived neurotrophic growth factor that helps boost neuroplasticity, which is the brain's capacity to shapeshift and migrate, and also enables the brain to manufacture new brain cells. Older brain cells may be retained while new ones are formed when there is a sufficient supply of BDNF, which means the brain will keep expanding because of the new cells that are arriving and remain healthy.

According to research, more especially when it has to do with synapses (where the neurotransmitter move from cell to cell), an Alkaline diet helps boost brain-derived neurotrophic growth factor. Diet following the 80/20 rule was demonstrated to raise the levels of brain-derived neurotrophic growth factor, by roughly 50-400% according to the study undertaken.

We now understand the relevance of nutrition to BDNF as far as the synapses are concerned. The neural plasticity through the food is increased substantially, which in turn helps to manage our mood better. That is, the strengthening or weakening of the synapse allows you to be in a moment of happiness or dread by modifying your mood accordingly.

What this method accomplishes for you according to common understanding is to assist you shift your mood and be reactive at the moment. You may be more concentrated when you want to be since you are in power of your attitude. You will be able to simply adapt in the moment. Your BDNF expression rises as your brain-derived neurotrophic growth factor rises, resulting in the synthesis and protection of more brain cells and providing your mind with all the tools it needs to maintain and recycle old cells by impacting cells on a genetic level (i.e. your DNA).

It also aids in the generation of growth hormone and serotonin in the body. A larger amount of growth hormone is considered a benefit in both men and women since it helps the brain renew much faster, and a research revealed an up to 4,000% rise in growth hormone levels. Growth hormones have a significant role in weight reduction and other aspects of health.

The diet helps in preventing osteoporosis

Osteoporosis is a condition that affects both men and women, particularly the elderly. Women who have passed menopause are most vulnerable. Osteoporosis is a major risk factor for bone fractures and the leading cause of fractured bones in the elderly. Another source of calcium insufficiency is this disorder.

The minerals present in the Dr. Sebi' diet have a similar effect on osteoporosis as they do on back pain. Though there is no scientific evidence to back this up, proponents of the alkaline diet claim that it reduces the amount of calcium lost in urine, lowering the risk of osteoporosis.

A number of fruits and vegetables have a unique method of boosting bone health, and alkaline diets low in protein are high in these items.

Sebi's diet improves your growth hormone levels

According to some data, increased growth hormone levels promote better brain functioning, notably memory and cognition, as well as enhanced heart health and even overall quality of life. Although there is no definite evidence relating an alkaline diet to increased growth hormone levels, several research suggest that rectifying a very acidic environment with specialised supplements such as bicarbonate can improve alkalinity.

Taking the diet helps you fighting fatigue

If you've been feeling weary recently, it might be because you've been eating too much acidic food. If all you consume is acidic food, too much of it might reduce your oxygen supply, and your body will no longer hold on to nutrients as readily even if you are receiving enough rest since the hydrogen potential in your body is uneven.

Consuming healthy green foods like cucumber, avocado, spinach, and broccoli on a daily basis helps alkalize your tissue, blood, and stem cell structure. Also, due to its high mineral concentration and pH of 8.5, alkaline water can assist improve the potential of hydrogen in your body.

Makes your teeth stronger

The dreadful impact of an acidic diet on one's teeth by burning away the protective enamel layer, leaving the teeth defenceless against hazardous acidic chemicals due to the teeth's already low pH value. Fruits and vegetables aid in the slowing of erosion.

Improves the body's ability to fight off infections (enhances immune system)

A robust immune system makes you less ill and more resistant to disease. According to one study, the Alkaline diet has been demonstrated to strengthen the immune system by taking into account an individual diet, especially how the stem cells regenerate. According to the study's findings, the Alkaline diet decreased white blood cells, causing the body to make less white blood cells and more stem cells, causing the body to develop better and more efficient cells.

With the formation of new cells and the release of old white blood cells, you will heal quickly overall.

The above-mentioned study discovered a lower level of Protein Kinase A (PKA), which aids in cell regeneration and allows them to produce new cells.

For those wishing to strengthen their immune system, the Alkaline diet has been demonstrated to lower insulin levels, which aids the immune system.

According to one study, a high level of insulin prevents T cells responsible for regulating inflammation and combating disease from completing their work properly. When your body's insulin level is high, your immune system suffers because T cells are no longer working at their best.

Because there are no insulin spikes when on a diet, T cells work at a greater level, thus increasing our immune system. Since you are on a diet, around 70% of your energy and blood flow to your stomach to digest the nutritious meal you have ingested, giving your body a chance to recuperate.

Our mental health and immune system cannot function without digestion. Our colon accounts for around 60% of our immune system, which implies that when we go on a diet, the entire body recovers, with a significant boost to the immune system.

Helps in longevity of life

There are several studies that illustrate the relevance of an alkaline diet in terms of increasing longevity. An alkaline diet aids Autophagy, a process of cell regeneration that involves removing old and weak cells and replacing them with younger and stronger ones. This, in turn, improves an individual's general well-being and lifespan.

Although no human studies have been conducted to support this idea, research demonstrate that lowering calories in animals by 30% to 40% boosts their lifetime, and that monkeys that ate less food but more on the Alkaline side lived longer.

This 25-year-long study, however, was later disproved by another study showing that it was not the case.

Although there is no genuine study to back up these assertions, it has been hypothesised that persons who ate less had a lower chance of disease, which might lead to longevity.

Helps decrease your stress

Stress is unavoidable wherever there is inflammation, as the two go hand in hand. A high degree of inflammation causes a high level of stress, and vice versa. Alkaline aids in stress relief by enhancing brain function. Your stress level will be reduced if your thinking is at its peak. Whether you are under pressure or not, the Alkaline diet helps with a healthier functioning brain, which eliminates any mental stress you may be experiencing.

Consult a doctor if you are under too much stress, since it may be caused by anything other than the Alkaline diet.

Dr. Sebi's Natural Detox Methods: A Step-by-Step Guide to Detoxification

The role of detoxification in the prevention and treatment of cancer

To have our cells and tissues regenerated, cleansed, and strengthened, one needs go through detoxification, which is made possible by alkalizing oneself through a raw food diet. This procedure removes acids and obstructions that create inflammation and prevent nourishment from reaching our bodily cells. Due to detoxification, cells are permitted to receive nutritional energy and appropriately discharge waste via cellular respiration, helping the body to repair itself.

According to research, it has been proved that an acidic (inflammatory, congestive, and putrefactive) diet including animal protein causes cancer. The congestive element of mucus is caused by its putrefactive and abrasive properties. Vaccinations, harmful chemicals, and hormones provided to or injected into these animals produce tissue toxicity within the body, causing inflammation to impair your immune system.

Consuming meat also causes a metabolic imbalance within the body. Because of the high levels of iron and phosphorus in the body, you begin to feel weakness and dehydration, which remove other useful minerals such as magnesium, calcium, and other essential electrolytes required by the body, making it hard to trace the presence of cancerous cells that emerge from these sources.

Chemotherapy and radiation do not work; instead, they worsen the problem by encouraging the malignant infection to spread to locations where cells have been damaged or killed by these therapies. Radiation destroys a cell's oxygen-carrying and utilisation factors. Glucose can still enter the cell through the cell membrane and cause fermentation and autointoxication.

The underlying element here is that over-acidity or inflammation, as well as the accumulation of cellular toxicity, produces cancer, resulting in the loss of cellular energy and function, and, in turn, the systematic loss of energy and health. As a result, our immune system becomes overworked. Because it is the tissue responsible for the synthesis of immune cells in a cancer patient, the Thymus gland (production site of T-cells) and bone marrow (production site of B-cells) become hypoactive.

Healthy lymphatic system is essential for a healthy body

90% of all disease processes originate in your lymphatic system, sometimes known as the "sewer system of the body," and a thorough grasp of it is advantageous. When your system is clogged and cannot correctly remove waste, it keeps the full waste product in the sewage system, resulting in inappropriate removal of metabolic or cellular wastes, as well as ingested metals and hazardous compounds. If these poisons are not removed, cellular death will result.

First, cleanse your lymphatic system so that your immune system can work more effectively, as the lymphatic system is an essential component of the immune system. It's important to note that the lymphatic system's secretion channels are your skin, kidney, and colon. A full or blocked septic system is just cleaned up; it is not removed.

Many people do not sweat adequately; their intestinal intestine walls are impacted; many have lost appropriate renal filtration; all of these are just indicators that the secretory channel is blocked due to its inability to allow waste to be properly removed. Because these wastes couldn't get out, they backed up to the lymphatic system, causing its nodes to widen, resulting in all kinds of lymphomas, throat cancer—especially after having the tonsils removed, non-estrogen types of breast cancer, colon, kidney, liver, and a slew of other issues because this process of always backing up the waste to the lymph system has been going on for years.

Your cells will begin to strengthen, and the toxic sludge that kills them will be removed by alkalinizing and purifying your fluids and tissues. This is why detoxification is essential in the treatment of cancer. You will start to feel more alive, energetic, and joyful.

There is no better method to restore and cleanse your body than via detoxification and cell regeneration with Dr. Sebi's diet and herbs. If you can only open your heart and accept responsibility for your health, you can do so much for your life and health.

Disorders and injuries related to the nervous system

Neurons are the greatest centres in the body, and they require the highest energy foods-fruits that work as an alkaline soil-to rejuvenate. Because fructose is a high energy simple sugar, it easily provides its energy to your cells. This approach is true for all neurological disorders, including Parkinson's, multiple sclerosis, asthma, and even Bell's palsy.

Every neurological deficit is preceded by an adrenal weakness. It is critical that the adrenal glands, along with the rest of the endocrine gland system, be increased for all neurological disorders, including traumas. This makes living on 100% raw food a must.

You may strengthen every cell in your body by following Dr. Sebi's diet and medicines. Herbal, brain, and nerve formulae of excellent quality are prescribed to further strengthen the nerve centres, spinal column, and brain tissue. Because the adrenal glands produce a large amount of our body's neurotransmitters and hormones, improving it is equally crucial.

In relation to neurological disorders and traumas, consider the thyroid/parathyroid. The parathyroid gland is required for optimal use. With Dr. Sebi's diet and proper calcium usage, your success is nearly certain.

The eradication of over-acidity, pain, cellulitis, tissue degradation, obesity, and urinary tract infections has substantially improved the quality of life of patients suffering from nerve injury, and they may enjoy total healing at the very best. Don't give up hope that the body can repair itself; it can.

The current food we eat has a high amount of toxin and acid, making it difficult for the body to repair owing to the high level of mucus, parasites, toxic chemicals, inflammation, and superfluous hormones. Avoid heated mucus-forming dairy foods, dead animal meat, processed sweets, and acidic fatty grains that serve no function other than to ruin the body. Abstaining from these meals allows you to rediscover the wonder of regeneration.

BOOK 3
Approved Food List

Dr. Sebi categorises food into six categories: raw food, live food, dead food, hybrid food, genetically modified food, and drugs. Dr. Sebi considers live and raw meals to be "electric foods" for the cells since they assist cure the body from the detrimental effects of acidic diet. He also believes that the other food classifications, such as pharmaceuticals, hybrid, dead, and genetically modified foods, should be avoided. Dr. Sebi's approved food list from the nutritional guidance is provided below;

FRUITS

Dr. Sebi has not allowed canned or seedless fruits.

- Tamarind
- Prunes
- Berries - All varieties.
- Apples
- Cantaloupe
- Currants
- Dates
- Cherries
- Grapes-seeded
- Limes (Key limes preferred with seeds)
- Plums
- Mango
- Melons-seeded
- Orange (Seville or sour preferred, difficult to find)
- Papayas
- Peaches
- Figs
- Pears
- Soft Jelly coconuts

- Prickly Pear (Cactus Fruit)

- Raisins -seeded

- Elderberries in any form. No Cranberries.

- Soursops (Latin or West Indian markets)

- Bananas -The smallest one or the Burro/midsize original banana Tamarind

VEGETABLES

- Okra

- Avocado

- Bell Peppers

- Chayote (Mexican squash)

- Dandelion Greens

- Green Banana

- Izote - cactus flower/cactus leaf

- Amaranth Greens

- Kale

- Lettuce- all, except iceberg

- Mushrooms - all, except Shitake

- Squash

- Nopales -Mexican Cactus

- Olives

- Onions

- Poke salad (Greens)

- Purslane (Verdolaga)

- Sea vegetables (wakame/Dulse/Arame/Hijiki/Nori)

- Tomato -cherry and plum only

- Wild Arugula

- Tomatillo
- Turnip Greens
- Cucumber
- Zucchini
- Watercress
- Garbanzo Beans

GRAINS

- Kamut
- Rye
- Wild Rice
- Fonio
- Quinoa
- Spelt
- Tef
- Amaranth

NATURAL HERBAL TEAS

- Chamomile
- Anise
- Tila
- Elderberry
- Allspice
- Fennel
- Ginger
- Burdock
- Raspberry

NUTS AND SEED (Includes Nut and Seed Butters)

- Brazilian Nuts
- Raw Sesame Seeds
- Raw Sesame "Tahini" Butter
- Walnuts
- Hemp Seeds

OILS

- Avocado Oil
- Grapeseed Oil
- Olive Oil (uncooked)
- Sesame Oil
- Hempseed Oil
- Coconut Oil (uncooked)

SWEET FLAVORS

SPICES AND SEASONINGS

- Date Sugar
- 100% Pure Agave Syrup (from cactus)

MILD FLAVORS

- Tarragon
- Bay Leaf
- Dill
- Parsley
- Oregano
- Thyme
- Basil

- Savoury

- Sweet Basil

- Cloves

SALTY FLAVORS

- Powdered Granulated Seaweed (Kelp/Dulce/Nori Has- "Sea Taste")

- Pure Sea Salt

PUNGENT AND SPICY FLAVORS

- Sage

- Coriander (Cilantro)

- Achiote

- Cayenne (African Bird Pepper)

- Onion Powder

- Habanero

BOOK 4
7 Day Meal Plan

DAY 1

BREAKFAST

BOWLS MADE WITH PLANT BASED QUINOA

This easy and delicious recipe for quinoa dish is very filling, very tasty, and above all very easy to prepare. If you like, this would be an excellent lunch or dinner recipe for you.

Which ingredients do you use to make this recipe?

Approximately one cup of cooked quinoa

1 or 2 greens that have been approved

Approximately two cups of chopped vegetables that have been approved

You will need one tablespoon of grapeseed oil for this recipe

What is the best way to prepare quinoa bowls that are plant-based?

This recipe starts with heating a large pan containing a tablespoon of grapeseed oil over medium-high heat, and then sautéing the sliced vegetables until they are tender.

As soon as you have cooked the quinoa, add in the fresh greens, quinoa flakes, and vegetables.

Afterwards, season it with cayenne pepper and sea salt according to your taste.

LUNCH

DR. SEBI'S MANGO SALAD

Having a mango salad is not a difficult or time-consuming task, and if you prepare it properly, it will be fresh and bright. If you start your 7 days of meal preparation with this salad, you will not be missing any meals, but you will be more committed to completing the program.

The ingredients that are used to make the recipe are as follows:

- 2 Mangoes
- Cayenne Pepper and Sea Salt
- ¼ Red Onion
- 1 key Lime
- ¼ Cup Cherry Tomatoes

- ½ Green Bell Pepper
- ½ Seeded Cucumber

Mango Salad - How do you prepare it?

The first thing you need to do when preparing a mango salad is to chop the mangoes, red onions, and cherry tomatoes into tiny cubes before you prepare the rest of the salad ingredients.

Then, you need to finely chop the bell pepper, cucumber, and seeds together.

In a mini bowl, combine all of the ingredients and squeeze the juice of one key lime over the salad. Then, mix all the ingredients together and place in a serving dish.

Place the chicken in a bowl, season it with pepper and salt, and place it in the fridge for 20 minutes, so that it can marinate.

It is now time to serve your salad and enjoy your meal.

DINNER

BASIL AVOCADO PASTA SALAD

The basil leaves of this combination have a very high nutritional value. They contain antioxidants that help to prevent the development of diseases as well as act as stress-busters.

The ingredients requires are as follow:

An avocado that has been chopped

Fresh basil leaves chopped into 1 cup

Cherry tomatoes, cut in half, 1 pint.

Key Lime Juice in the amount of one tablespoon

In a small bowl, add 1 teaspoon of Agave Syrup and mix well

¼ Cup of Olive Oil

You will need four cups of cooked spelt pasta (any pasta that has been approved by Dr. Sebi is fine)

Below, I will show you how to prepare basil avocado pasta salad.

Put the cooked pasta in a large mixing basin.

Then, add the basil, avocado, and tomatoes and thoroughly combine until all ingredients are well combined.

In a small mixing bowl, combine the lime, oil, sea salt, and agave syrup.

Pour it over the spaghetti and keep swirling until it is thoroughly combined.

DAY 2

BREAKFAST

KAMUT BREAKFAST PORRIDGE

Fill a large mixing bowl halfway with cooked spaghetti.

Then, add the basil, avocado, and tomatoes and thoroughly blend until everything is completely incorporated.

Combine the lime, oil, sea salt, and agave syrup in a small mixing dish.

Pour it over the spaghetti and continue to swirl until fully mixed.

Ingredients required for making it are:

Kamut flour (one cup or seven ounces)

A total of 3¾ cups of homemade walnut milk or coconut milk that is in the form of soft jelly

A tablespoon of coconut oil can be used instead of the palm oil

Sea salt (approximately ½ tablespoons)

Agave syrup 4 tablespoons

Kamut Breakfast Porridge:

How to Prepare it?

In a high-speed food processor or blender, grind the Kamut until you have 114 cups of cracked Kamut.

In a medium saucepan, combine the walnut or coconut milk, cracked Kamut, and sea salt.

Allow it to boil over high heat for approximately 10 minutes, then gradually decrease the heat from high to low and simmer, stirring regularly to get the desired thickness.

Remove from the heat after 10 minutes and whisk in the agave syrup and coconut oil.

If desired, top the dish with fresh fruits and enjoy your Kamut porridge.

LUNCH

STEWED OKRA AND TOMATOES WILD RICE

In addition to being a very affordable dish, it is also very easy to prepare. You can mix it with either wild rice or quinoa for more variety.

Ingredients that you will need:

Fresh Okra, 2 cups of it

You will need 1 cup of cherry tomatoes for this recipe

Onion, medium size, 1

Avocado oil - 1 Tablespoon (60 ml)

Water from a fresh spring, ½ cups

Cayenne and sea salt

The best way to prepare stewed okra and tomatoes is to follow these steps:

Peel and dice the onion and cherry tomatoes.

Heat the avocado oil in a pan, then add the chopped onion. Allow to simmer until the onion is transparent.

When the onion becomes transparent, add the spring water and okra. Cook for around 10 minutes on low heat.

Add the chopped cherry tomatoes and simmer for about 20 minutes, or until the okra is tender.

Then season with pepper and sea salt to taste.

DINNER

DANDELION STRAWBERRY SALAD

Dandelion greens are very therapeutic and have long been used to cure a variety of diseases. Dandelion has been shown in current scientific studies to destroy germs and other microorganisms, as well as to have anti-cancer properties. To get the greatest flavour, combine it with savoury and sweet ingredients.

Ingredients you need to have to prepare this

You will need two teaspoons of grapeseed oil for this recipe

(Sliced) 1 medium red onion (medium size)

Approximately 10 ripe strawberries (sliced)

In a small bowl, add 2 tablespoons of key lime juice

Dandelion Greens - 4 cups

Sea Salt according to your taste

Dandelion Strawberry Salad:

How Do You Make It?

In a 12-inch nonstick frying pan, heat the grapeseed oil over medium heat to warm it up. Add the diced red onions and season with salt. Cook, stirring periodically, until the onions are soft, light brown, and approximately one-third the size they were when raw.

Toss the chopped strawberries with 1 teaspoon key lime juice in a small bowl. Wash the dandelion greens and dice them into desired sizes.

When the onions are almost done, add the remaining key lime juice to the pan. Cook for another minute or two, or until the sauce thickens enough to cover the onions. Take the onions out of the pan.

In a salad dish, combine the onions, greens, and strawberries with all of their juices, and season with sea salt.

DAY 3

BREAKFAST

GREEN DETOX SMOOTHIE AND JUICY PORTOBELLO BURGER

Green detox smoothie promotes the process of detoxification by removing toxic waste from the body. When coupled with a meaty Portobello mushroom burger, they make an amazing combination that will satiate you while also providing a health benefit.

Green Detox Smoothie

To prepare it, you will need these ingredients?

½ Burro Banana

½ Cup Ginger Tea

½ Cup of Soft Jelly Coconut Water

2 – 3 Tablespoon of Key Lime Juice

¼ Cup of Blueberries

1 Cup Romaine Lettuce

How Do You Make a Green Detox Smoothie?

Make the tea and set it aside to cool.

Using a blender, combine all of the ingredients.

Juicy Portobello Burger

What are the ingredients?

1 Avocado (Sliced)

3 Tablespoon of Olive Oil

1 Tablespoon of Dried Oregano

2 Tablespoon of Dried Basil

2 Large Portobello Mushroom Caps

1 Tomato (Sliced)

1 Cup Purslane

How to Prepare Juicy Portobello Burger?

As if cutting a bun, cut the mushroom stems at approximately 12 of the mushroom top.

In a small mixing bowl, combine the onion powder, olive oil, cayenne pepper, basil, and oregano.

To avoid sticking, brush the foil with grapeseed oil before placing the mushroom caps on it.

Allow the marinade to sit for about 10 minutes after pouring it over the mushroom cap with a big spoon.

Preheat the oven to 425°F before placing the mushroom in it to bake for about 10 minutes, checking regularly to see if it is done before flipping it to bake for another 10 minutes.

Serve by placing the bottom of the mushroom cap on a plate and garnishing it with your favourite toppings before covering it with the upper section of the mushroom cap.

LUNCH

MAGIC GREEN FELAFEL

The magic green falafel recipe resists frying and is an alkaline electric food with a fantastic flavour. It is incredibly simple and quick to make, and you will appreciate it.

What are the Ingredients?

2/3 Cup of Fresh Basil

2 Cups of Dry Garbanzo Beans (Chickpeas)

1/3 Cup of Red Bell Pepper (Chopped)

1/4 Teaspoon of Oregano

1/2 Cup of Fresh Dill

1 Teaspoon of Sea Salt

1/2 Cup of Garbanzo Bean Flour

1 Large Onions (Chopped)

Grapeseed or Avocado Oil for Frying

How Do You Make Magical Green Falafel?

The first step in making magic green falafel is to cook the chickpeas until they are soft, then drain and rinse the beans.

In a food processor, combine the chickpeas and the remaining ingredients (the red bell pepper, onion, sea salt, oregano, flour, and fresh herbs.)

Pulse the ingredients until they make a coarse meal or are finely chopped. Scrape down the sides of the food processor and continue pulsing until the mixture is fine. Taste it and adjust the seasoning as needed.

Transfer the mixture to a large mixing basin with your hands, then shape into thick discs or tiny balls and wrap in parchment paper. Allow at least 1 hour to chill in the refrigerator.

Fill a big pan approximately 1 inch deep with oil. Cook the oil for 5-7 minutes on low heat. The Magic Green Falafels should then be deep fried for around 2-3 minutes on each side.

DINNER

THE GRILLED ROMAINE LETTUCE SALAD

This meal is a tasty alternative to the typical lettuce salad. The basis is grilled romaine lettuce, which gives it a distinct flavour.

What exactly are the ingredients?

4 Small Heads Romaine Lettuce (Rinsed)

1 Tablespoon of Red Onion (Finely Chopped)

1 Tablespoon of Key Lime Juice.

1 Tablespoon of Agave Syrup

4 Tablespoons of Olive Oil

1 Tablespoon of Fresh Basil (Chopped)

Sea Salt and Cayenne Pepper to taste

How to Prepare Grilled Romaine Lettuce Salad?

Place the lettuce halves on a large nonstick skillet. Allow the lettuce to grill without adding oil to the pan, turning it regularly to check its colour; after it is brown on both sides, remove the pan from the heat.

Place the lettuce on a large plate to chill.

In a mixing bowl, combine the ingredients (agave syrup, red onion, key lime juice, olive oil, and fresh basil), then season with salt and pepper to taste.

Place the grilled lettuce on a serving dish and top with the dressing.

Enjoy your meal.

DAY 4

BREAKFAST

GREEN PANCAKE

One big issue that folks who follow plant-based diets encounter is a lack of protein; people frequently worry about losing muscle and other such things. With garbanzo bean as its major component, this Green Pancake is naturally full of protein and includes enough minerals and fibre to build up the body.

What are the Ingredients?

1 tbsp of your preferred nut butter for added protein (homemade walnut, homemade tahini, or Brazil nut butter)

½ Teaspoon of Sea Salt

½ Cup of Spring Water

¼ Cup of Blueberries

½ Cup of Chickpea Flour

1 Handful of Amaranth Green

1 Tablespoon of Agave Syrup

How Do You Make Green Pancakes?

To begin, combine all of the ingredients in a blender and mix until smooth. When adding water, be cautious since too much water may damage the food, making it less fluffy and perhaps not cooking properly.

Allow the mixed mixture to rest for 5-10 minutes. While it settles, prepare a nonstick pan and heat it on low heat.

Scoop the mixed mixture into a frying pan to make six tiny pancakes. The size is up to you; you may alternatively create three giant pancakes or 4-5 regular pancakes.

Allow them to simmer until you notice bubbles on the mixed mixture, they become fluffy, and they appear cooked around the edges. Then flip it over and cook for a few minutes.

After that, you may top it with burro banana, agave syrup, or blueberries and enjoy your meal.

LUNCH

ALKALINE MUSHROOM GRAVY

The alkaline mushroom gravy is made completely of plant-based ingredients.

So, here are the ingredients you would need.

1 Pinch each of Cayenne pepper and Sea Salt

2 Tablespoons of Finely Chopped Walnuts

½ Cup of Homemade Approved Vegetable Broth

1 cup mushrooms, thinly sliced (all types of mushrooms except for shiitake)

1½ Tablespoon of Amaranth or Spelt Flour

¼ of an Onion (Diced)

2 Tablespoon of Grapeseed Oil

1 Cup of Homemade Walnut Milk

½ Teaspoon of Fresh Thyme

Alkaline Mushroom Gravy: How to Make It

Cook on medium heat with the grapeseed oil in the pan you wish to use, either a saucepan or a cast-iron skillet. Then season with the onion, mushroom, and a touch of cayenne pepper and sea salt. Cook for about 3 - 4 minutes, or until the onion turns translucent.

Mix in the spelt flour and amaranth until thoroughly combined. Then cook for another minute.

12 cup at a time, gradually combine the homemade vegetable broth and walnut milk. Then season with cayenne pepper and sea salt to taste. Cook until it thickens, stirring constantly over low heat. You may taste and adjust the seasoning to your liking.

You may now add the walnuts and thoroughly mix them up. Make sure it's on low heat, and you may add more walnut milk to thin it down if it's too thick.

It goes well with plant-based biscuits or bread prepared with flour derived from any of the allowed grains.

DINNER

ZUCCHINI BREAD PANCAKE

Here are the ingredients you need to have.

2 Cups of Homemade Walnut Milk

¼ Cup of Mashed Burro Banana

2 Cups of Spelt or Kamut Flour

1 Cup of Finely Shredded Zucchini

½ Cup of Chopped Walnuts

2 Tablespoon of Date Sugar

What Is the Best Way to Make Zucchini Bread Pancakes?

Combine the flour and date sugar in a large mixing bowl.

Combine the mashed burro banana and walnut milk in a mixing bowl. To ensure that no dry mix has been stuck to the bottom of the bowl, thoroughly whisk it.

Combine the shredded zucchini and walnuts separately.

Heat the grapeseed oil in a skillet or griddle over medium-high heat.

Pour the mixed ingredients into the skillet to make your pancakes. Cook for an additional 4 to 5 minutes on each side.

Your meal is finished; serve with agave syrup to enjoy.

DAY 5

BREAKFAST

ZOODLES WITH AVOCADO PEAR

Sea Salt to taste

What are the ingredients?

½ Cup of Walnuts

½ Cup of Water

2 Large Zucchinis

2 Cups of Basil

2 Avocados

24 Sliced Cherry Tomatoes

4 Tablespoons of Key Lime Juice

How to Prepare Zoodles with Avocado Pear?

To prepare the zucchini noodles, use a spiralizer or peeler.

Blend all of the ingredients, except the cherry tomatoes, in a blender until smooth.

Mix up the avocado sauce, cherry tomatoes, and noodles in a mixing dish.

Serve your lunch and enjoy it.

LUNCH

CLASSIC HOMEMADE HUMMUS

This traditional homemade hummus recipe is a must-have in any home; it is a staple item that can be produced quickly and effortlessly. It's incredibly creamy, smooth, tasty, and delicious. When you're in a rush or running late for work, this is an excellent breakfast option.

What are the ingredients?

A Dash of Onion Powder

Sea Salt to taste

2 Tablespoons Key Lime Juice

1 Cup of Cooked Chickpeas

2 Tablespoons Olive Oil

1/3 Cup Homemade Tahini Butter

How to Make Traditional Homemade Hummus

Simply combine all of the ingredients in a high-powered blender and mix.

Serve your food and enjoy it.

DINNER

HEALTHY FRIED RICE

With this dish, you can say good-by to Chinese take-out for a tasty fried rice meal. All you have to do is follow these easy instructions and you will be healthy.

Ingredients involved in preparing it:

½ Cup of Zucchini

Cayenne Pepper and Sea Salt to taste

½ Cup of Bell Peppers

1 Cup of Wild Rice or Quinoa

¼ Onion

1 Tablespoon of Grapeseed Oil½

Cup of Mushrooms

How Can I Make Healthy Fried Rice?

The first step is to per-boil the rice after thoroughly cleaning it.

Then cut all of the ingredients (bell pepper, mushroom, zucchini, and onion (cubed)) into slices.

Heat the grapeseed oil in a frying pan, then add the onion and cook until it is browned.

Cook for about 5 minutes with all of the cut veggies. However, make sure they don't grow too soft.

Cook the cooked rice until it has become brown.

You may now serve and enjoy your dinner.

DAY 6

BREAKFAST

WILD RICE MUSHROOM

What are the ingredients?

2 wild rice and long grain mix six-pound packages

½ Cup Chopped Fresh Flat-Leaf Parsley

12 oz. Assorted Fresh Mushrooms (Sliced and Trimmed)

½ Cup Marsala

3 Tablespoon of Grapeseed Oil

1 Large Sweet Onion (Diced)

¼ Teaspoon Salt

How to Cook Wild Rice Mushroom

The first step is to per-boil the rice after thoroughly cleaning it.

Heat the grapeseed oil in a large pan over medium heat.

Then add the onion and cook for 7 minutes, or until it begins to brown.

Cook for 4 to 5 minutes, or until the mushroom softens, with the mushroom and salt.

Cook for 3 minutes, or until the liquid is absorbed, after adding the marsala.

Combine the mushroom and parsley in a bowl and pour over the rice.

Serve and enjoy your dinner.

LUNCH

DETOX SALAD BURRITOS AND DETOX SMOOTHIE

Ingredients needed

Cayenne Pepper and Sea salt to taste

2 cups wild arugula or any other grain allowed

1 Cup of Cooked Chickpeas (Garbanzo Beans)

1 Tablespoon of Key Lime Juice

2 Cups of Cherry Tomatoes

1 Tablespoon of Homemade Raw Sesame Tahini Butter

4 Kamut Flour Tortillas

Detox Salad Burritos: How to Make Them

To make the dressing, combine the key lime juice and raw sesame tahini butter in a small cup and put aside.

Then, in a large mixing dish, combine chickpeas, wild arugula, and cherry tomatoes. Cover this mixture with the dressing and place it in the refrigerator to allow the flavours to blend.

Warm up the Kamut flour tortillas on a large griddle or skillet over low heat until they become flexible.

After filling the tortillas with the salad, season with the cayenne pepper and sea salt. You may then roll it up.

Serve your lunch and enjoy it.

DINNER

MUSHROOM, VEGAN CHEESE, AND ALMOND RISOTTO

Ingredients content:

24 Ounce of Vegetable broth

1½ Cups of Arborio Rice

1½ Tablespoons of Butter

½ Cup Grated Vegan Cheese

2 Tablespoon Sliced Almonds

Sea Salt and Cayenne Pepper

8 Ounce of Baby Bella Mushrooms (Sliced)

How to Prepare Risotto with Mushrooms, Vegan Cheese, and Almonds

To begin, pour the vegetable broth into a pot and slowly heat it.

Melt your butter in a medium saucepan over medium-low heat. Then add the cooked rice and lightly toast it. Allow it to sit for 2 minutes, or until the colour shifts from pure white to slightly off white. The rice should be stirred regularly.

Pour in just enough vegan broth to cover the rice. Allow it to cook on low heat.

Heat the remaining butter on a griddle or pan over medium heat. Then add the mushrooms and toss to coat evenly with the butter. Season with cayenne pepper and sea salt to taste. Allow the mushrooms to cook for about 8 minutes, or until they are all brown, and keep warm.

Stir the rice regularly with a wooden spoon. Pour in enough liquid to thoroughly cover the rice and leave to simmer until it has absorbed the original stock.

You may now toast the almonds in an oven for 1 - 2 minutes at 350 degrees Fahrenheit, or until they turn golden. Set aside the toasted almond.

The cooked rice may require a third or even fourth addition of liquid. The goal is for the rice to be cooked but not overcooked. It should be chewy rather than mushy. To determine whether a fourth broth is necessary, taste the rice before and after adding the third broth.

When the rice is fully cooked, toss in the cheese and mushrooms. Then season with cayenne pepper and sea salt to taste.

You may serve it with the roasted almonds on top and enjoy your supper.

DAY 7

BREAKFAST

ASIAN SESAME DRESSING AND NOODLES

Ingredients needed:

Asian Sesame Dressing

2 Teaspoons Gluten-Free Tamari

½ Teaspoon of Lemon

2 Tablespoons of Sesame Butter (Tahini)

1 Freshly Squeezed Clove Garlic (Minced)

½ Teaspoon of Liquid Coconut Nectar (Coconut Secrets Brand)

Noodles Salad

1 Tablespoon of Raw Sesame Seeds (Toppings)

1 Scallion (Chopped)

Red Bell Pepper and Carrot (Sliced)

How to Make Asian Sesame Dressing and Noodles

You may choose between zucchini and kelp noodles. If you're using kelp noodles, soak them in warm water for 10 minutes to remove the package liquid and soften and separate them. If you're making zucchini noodles, though, you'll need a vegetable peeler or spiralizer.

Place all of the dressing ingredients in a mixing bowl and well combine with a spoon.

Then, stir together the Asian sesame dressing with the scallions and noodles.

Serve garnished with sesame seeds on top.

LUNCH

FAT-FREE PEACH MUFFINS

This meal is really beneficial to your gallbladder. Its low fat content aids in the reduction and management of gallstone symptoms. This dinner is not only healthy, but it is also really flavorful and wonderful.

Ingredients required:

2 Cups of Spelt Flour

2 Large Peaches about 2 Cups (Chopped)

2 Tablespoons of Warm Spring Water

1 Tablespoon of Agave Syrup

2 Teaspoon of Key Lime Juice

1½ Teaspoons of Mashed Burro Banana

½ Cup of Date Sugar

¼ Teaspoon Salt

2 Tablespoons of Chopped Walnuts

1¼ Cups of Homemade Walnut Milk

Procedure to Make Fat-Free Peach Muffins

To begin, preheat your oven to 400°F. Then, prepare your muffin pan by spreading some grapeseed oil into it.

Peel the skin off the peaches (if using a really ripe peach, the skin will come off easily; if not, immerse the peaches in boiling water for approximately 30 seconds, peel when it cools, and remove the pit).

You may combine the walnut milk and key lime juice with the burro banana.

In a large mixing bowl, combine the sea salt, date sugar, and flour.

Continue stirring while adding the liquid components and ensuring adequate mixing (batter will be thick). Fold the peaches well and spread them evenly over the batter.

Fill the muffin to about 12 inch from the top and level the top of the muffin. Chopped walnuts can be put on top if desired.

Bake for 15 to 20 minutes, or until a toothpick inserted into the centre comes out clean. Allow the muffins to cool completely before serving.

DINNER

DR. SEBI's MUSHROOM RISOTTO

This dish is creamy, thick, and flavorful. This is going to be the finest mushroom you've ever had.

Ingredients needed

Cayenne Pepper to taste 4 Mushrooms

1 Tablespoon Grapeseed Oil

4 cups vegetable broth (homemade) (from any of the approved vegetables)

2 Cups of wild Rice

Sea Salt to taste

How to Make Dr. Sebi's Mushroom Risotto

Place the grapeseed oil in a large saucepan over medium heat.

Place the onions and mushrooms in the saucepan and simmer for 5 - 7 minutes, or until the mushrooms are browned and all of the liquid has evaporated. Stir and combine occasionally.

Allow the cooked rice to boil for one minute.

Add the veggie broth, cayenne pepper, and sea salt. Then, cover it tightly and cook it for 2 hours 45 minutes on low heat or 1 hour 15 minutes on high heat, or until the rice softens.

Serve your lunch and enjoy it.

Dr. Sebi's diet has increased in favour among the younger population for many years. This new trend is gaining traction as a result of the present generation's unhealthy eating habits. They have access to a plethora of quick meals, many of which include hazardous minerals that can lead to long-term problems such as cancer. As a result, it is not surprising that individuals are becoming increasingly interested in natural ways to cleanse their system. As a result, there is a high demand for Dr. Sebi's Alkaline Diet.

The 3-step approach for detoxing your body naturally;

Step 1

This alkaline diet is a theory that is not entirely supported by research, but it is thought that an alkaline technique provides a barrier against germs. Various plant-based diets have been developed on this premise to lower the level of acidity in the body. Aside from this common sense premise, it is common known that meals not on Dr. Sebi's lists have a long term effect on the body; this feature has been scientifically proven. The alkaline diet is primarily vegan and has several drawbacks.

Step 2

Dr. Sebi's alkaline diet has a rigorous food list that must be followed in order to achieve the best results. Dairy items, canned foods, seedless fruits, processed foods, and synthetic foods are all forbidden. Although these meals are widely available, they are not healthy to consume on a daily basis. Alkaline diets advocate for more natural foods with lower acidic content, such as vegetables, fruits with seeds, and some grains, oils, teas, and spices, among others.

Step 3

All of these diets have been thoroughly researched, and a weekly food plan has been created to help you. The meal was divided into three meals: breakfast, lunch, and supper, with morning being lighter foods and lunch and dinner being heavier depending on your preferences.

Following this instruction will result in a stronger and healthier system. Even if you miss a day, you can always make it up because the aim is to get your system completely operational. These meals are not only delicious, but they may also help revive your body's organs, particularly the kidney.

BOOK 5
Dr. Sebi Treatment and Cures

How to Cure Cancer, Diabetes, Lupus, Herpes, HIV, Hair Loss, and Other Diseases Using Dr. Sebi's Alkaline Diet

Introduction

Herbs and natural foods have been utilised since time immemorial, and they have shown to be healthy and effective in the treatment of chronic illnesses such as diabetes and mental disease. To begin, we must define herbs and examine some old uses, as well as their makeup. Herbs are versatile plants that have fragrant components that are used in cooking and medicine.

History

Herb use may be traced back to 5000 BCE, proving that Sumerians used plants for medicinal purposes. The legendary physicians were well-known for using around 100 components in the formulation of certain herbal treatments. Some plants also contain phytochemicals that may be harmful to the body. Furthermore, certain herbs have impacts on the body when they are digested, such as when they are used to spice food, and other herbs can be dangerous when consumed in excess. Hypericum perforatum or Piper methysticum, for example, is used to treat stress and sadness. Nonetheless, an excess of these herbs may cause difficulties, so they must be used with caution.

When used with certain prescription medicines, further issues may occur.

Herbs have long been utilised as the foundation of Chinese natural medicine in general, dating back to the first century AD, and Ayurvedic treatments in India are likewise founded on herbs. In Western culture, plant healing is founded in the Hippocratic (Greek) theory of healing elements, which is based on a metaphor for replenishing quaternary components.

Renowned Western herbalists include Avicenna (Persian), Galen (Roman), Paracelsus (German-Swiss), Culpeper (UK), and a botanist from America in the 19th/early 20th centuries (John Milton Scudder, Harvey W.). John Uri Lloyd). Modern medicine is derived from raw herbal medicines, and certain capsules are still extracted as components fractionated/isolated from herbal raw materials and then refined to pharmaceutical standards.

Some plants contain psychoactive components, which were employed for a variety of secular and recreational reasons in the early Holocene era with the help of humans. People in northern Peruvian civilization have eaten the leaves and strong extracts of the cannabis and coca plants for more than 8,000 years, while the usage of marijuana herbs as a chemical that affects the mind goes back to the first century AD. in China and North Africa.

Indigenous Australians created "shrub medicine" using only plants that were readily available to them. Because of their seclusion, these firms' medications affect considerably fewer ailments than western diseases, which declined during colonisation. Coughs, diarrhoea, fever, and headaches have all been treated using herbs like as peppermint, rosemary, and eucalyptus.

Naturally Cleanse with Herbs and Product

Herbs have inherent healing properties. Dr. Sebi has devised a rigorous plant-based diet to assist extract the most benefit from these plants. Dr. Sebi thinks that ailments are caused by mucous and acidity. He also demonstrated that consuming certain foods and avoiding others might naturally cleanse the body, resulting in an alkaline condition that can help lower the likelihood of illness.

According to Dr. Sebi, illnesses can only exist in an acidic environment. The diet's main goal is to get the body to an alkaline condition in order to prevent or eradicate illness.

How to Stick to the Diet

There are several principles to follow in Dr. Sebi's nutritional guidance to attain the greatest outcomes.

Eat just the foods in the list.

1 gallon of natural spring water every day

Animal products, hybrid meals, and alcohol should be avoided.

Avoid using a microwave since it will "destroy your food."

Avoid canned fruits and seeds.

The Dr. Sebi diet includes the following components:

Avocados, kale, bell peppers, and wild arugula are among the vegetables.

Apples, bananas, dates, and Seville oranges are among the fruits.

Grains including rye, spelt, wild rice, and quinoa

Avocado, hempseed, coconut, and olive oils are examples of oils, however Dr. Sebi cautions against using the latter two in cooking.

Hemp and raw sesame seeds, tahini butter, and walnuts are examples of nuts and seeds.

Herbal teas, such as chamomile, fennel, and ginger teas

Natural sweeteners like agave syrup and date sugar

What Are the Advantages?

Despite the fact that there is no scientific evidence to support the Dr. Sebi diet, several studies suggest that a plant-based diet may maintain and enhance health. There are no dangers to be concerned about.

The following are some of the health benefits of plant-based diets:

Weight reduction – According to a 2015 study, a vegan eating plan resulted in more weight loss than other, less stringent diets. After 6 months on a vegan diet, the participants dropped up to 7.5% of their body weight.

Appetite manipulation – A 2016 study of younger male participants revealed that they felt more full and snug after eating a plant-based dinner with peas and beans rather than a meat-based one.

Changing the microbiome — The term "microbiome" refers to the bacteria in the intestine. According to a 2019 study, a plant-based diet can improve the microbiome, resulting in a lower risk of illness. However, further study will be required to corroborate this.

Reduced illness risk - According to a 2017 study, a diet based only on herbs may lower the risk of heart disease by 40%, as well as the chance of developing metabolic syndrome and type 2 diabetes by half.

Natural food contains one of Dr. Sebi's requirements. He advises us to consume more edible and natural foods instead of manufactured stuff.

Dr. Sebi's Products

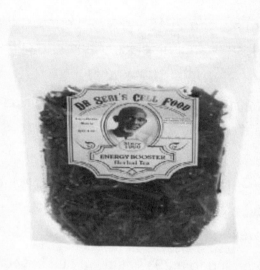

Dr. Sebi's Energy Booster Tea

Dr. Sebi's Energy Booster tea is specifically designed to maximise your body's energy levels. It raises your body's iron levels, which allows more oxygen to be carried in the haemoglobin of red blood cells throughout the body, allowing the cells to create energy. Muicle has been utilised for its antioxidant qualities, detoxifying capabilities, and effectiveness as a blood cleanser. Even today, many people use this potent herb as part of their daily regimen to feel more energised than ever! Directions: 2 cups purified water, plus 112 tablespoons Dr. Sebi's Energy Booster Tea Cook for around 15 minutes. Allow to cool before straining. Should be consumed twice day.

Ingredients:

- Muicle

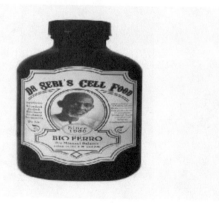

Bio Ferro

Bio Ferro combines the best nutrients to deliver the most potent and effective method of nourishing and purifying the blood. Yellow dock root (Rumex Crispus) is a natural plant that is used to treat indigestion as a bitter digestive medication. Yellow dock root is an all-purpose blood cleanser and detoxifier, particularly for the liver. Yellow dock root promotes bile production, which assists digestion, particularly fat digestion. It can promote bowel motions, which can help cleanse clogged intestines. It also raises the rate of urine, which aids in the removal of pollutants.

Ingredients:

- Cocolmeca
- Chaparral
- Burdock Root
- Elderberry
- Yellow dock

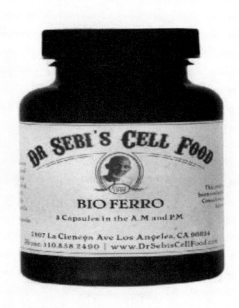

Bio Ferro Capsules

Bio Ferro pills have the appropriate components to nourish and cleanse the blood in the most potent and effective way. Chaparral (Larrea Tridentate) is regarded as a potent antioxidant. Chaparral has been utilised by Native Americans to cure a range of ailments, including respiratory sickness, chickenpox, snake bites, and arthritic pain. Chaparral is a fantastic medicine for treating liver health, cleaning the blood, boosting immunity, decreasing weight, and general well-being due to its potent antioxidant capabilities. It's also used to treat digestive issues including cramps and gas, as well as respiratory issues.

Ingredients:

- Yellowdock

- Burdock

- Chaparral

- Nopal

- Nettle

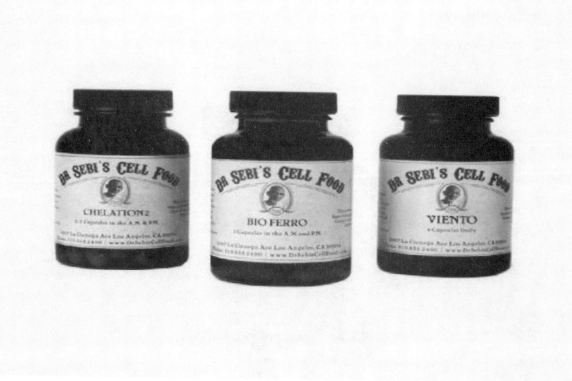

Small Cleansing Package

Chelation2, Bio Ferro, and Viento are included in the little cleaning pack. This cleaning pack was created to cleanse and nourish your body on a cellular level. This bundle aids in the removal of mucus, poisons, and acids from the body. It will also nourish and cleanse the blood, restoring the entire body to its original state. This is no longer a treatment plan.

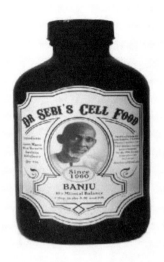

Banju

Banju was created using a one-of-a-kind blend of potent substances. This tonic was designed to boost the brain and neurological system. Elderberry is a huge shrub or small tree that may grow up to 30 feet tall in either wet or dry soil in a sunny position.

Ingredients:

- Bugleweed
- Blue Vervain
- Elderberry
- •Burdock Root
- Valerian Root

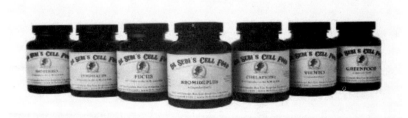

Booster

The booster package adds components to your body's revitalising process. This mechanism strengthens the intercellular repair and cleansing process even further.

Products Included (7 products):

- Bromide Plus Capsules
- Green Food
- Lymphalin
- Fucus Liquid
- Bio Ferro Capsules
- Chelation 2
- Viento

Dr. Sebi's Immune Support Herbal Tea

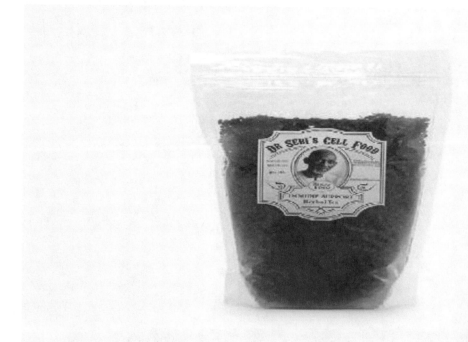

Dr. Sebis Cell Food is pleased to offer an immune-boosting herbal tea with the natural antioxidant elderberry. Elderberry has antiviral and cancer-fighting qualities and can help decrease swelling of the mucous membrane lining, particularly the sinuses. Ideally, you should be able to boost your immune system.

Elderberry can also help with cholesterol, sore throats, coughs, colds, flu, bacterial and viral infections, and respiratory issues. It also helps to prevent autoimmune illnesses. Elderberry also includes flavonoids, which have antioxidant characteristics and can aid in the prevention of cell damage.

Directions:

Boil two glasses of purified water and add 1½ teaspoons of Dr. Sebi's herbal immune booster tea. Allow it to boil for 15 minutes. Allow to cool before straining. It must be consumed twice day.

Ingredients:

- Elderberry

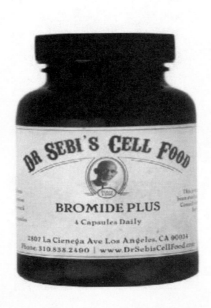

Bromide Plus Capsules

People with poor breath, lung illness, respiratory issues, and diarrhoea will benefit from it. Bromide Plus is a natural diuretic that also lowers hunger, controls the intestines, and aids the digestive system as a whole. Bromide Plus is safe to use throughout the digestive system. Bladderwrack (Fucus Vesiculous) is an alga found on the Pacific, Atlantic, and Baltic Sea coasts. It is the most important source of iodine. Bladderwrack has high levels of beta-carotene, bromine, potassium, alginic acid, and mannitol.

Ingredients:

- Irish Seamoss
- Bladderwrack

Eyewash

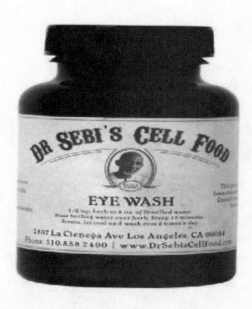

It functions as a natural eye nourisher and cleanser. Euphrasia (Eyebright) is used to treat a variety of eye conditions. It alleviates eye discomfort caused by blepharitis and conjunctivitis.

Ingredients:

- Eyebright

Green Food

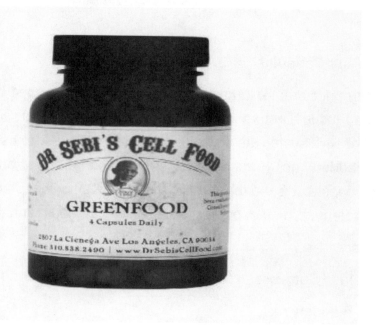

This is a multi-mineral component created from African plants that provides chlorophyll-rich fuel for the entire body. It improves overall good health and nutrition. Ortigia (Urtica Dioica) is a well-known anti-inflammatory herb that has been used to treat kidney disorders, urinary tract infections (enlarged prostate, nighttime urination, regular urination, painful urination, and irritable bladder), gastrointestinal tract disorders, locomotor system disorders, cardiovascular system, haemorrhage, influenza, rheumatism, and gout. It is also eco-friendly as a blood cleanser and for treating poor circulation. Ortiga has traditionally been used to treat hypersensitivity response symptoms, particularly hay fever.

Ingredients:

- Bladderwrack
- Tila
- Nettle
- Nopal

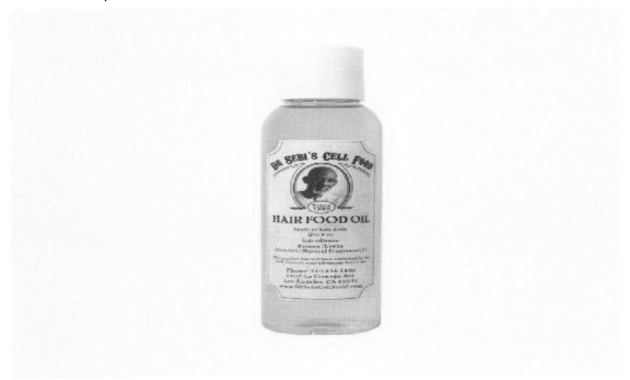

Hair Food Oil

It encourages hair development and is beneficial to the scalp. It is mild enough to use on a regular basis. Ingredients include:

Ingredients:

- Coconut Oil

- French Vanilla fragrance oil

- Batana

- Olive Oil

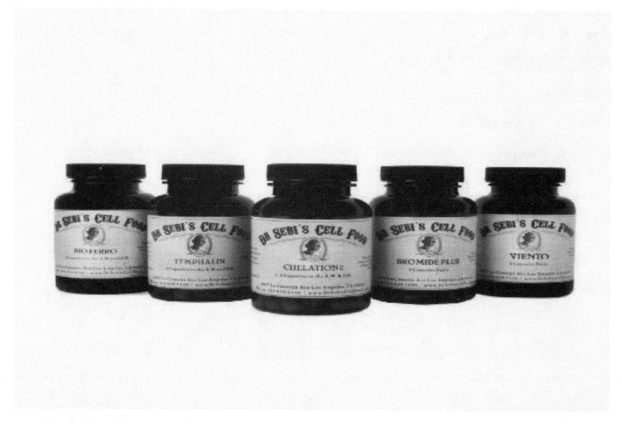

Support Package

The Support package guides your body through a healing process. This package is designed to provide inter-cellular repair and detoxification.

Products Included (5 products):

- Bio Ferro Capsules

- Lymphalin

- Viento

- Chelation 2

- Bromide Plus Capsules

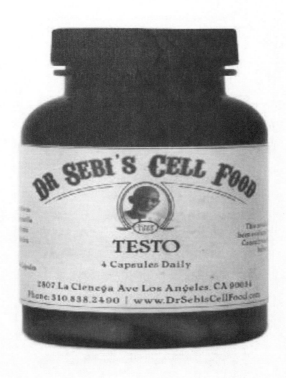

Testo

Testo is one of the world's natural boosters used to increase testosterone production in men. Dr. Sebi's unique mixture combines the correct herbs to create a potent synergy that boosts testosterone levels.

Benefits:

- It supports Male Hormonal Balance.
- It is a Natural Testosterone Booster.
- It provides strength.
- It promotes Endurance.
- It promotes Stamina.
- It improves Sexual Health.
- It increases Libido (Sexual Desire.)
- It promotes healthy blood flow to the male genitalia (Blood vessel tone and dilatation.)

Ingredients:

- Irish Seamoss
- Yohimbi
- Sarsaparilla
- Locust Bark
- Capadulla

Tooth Powder

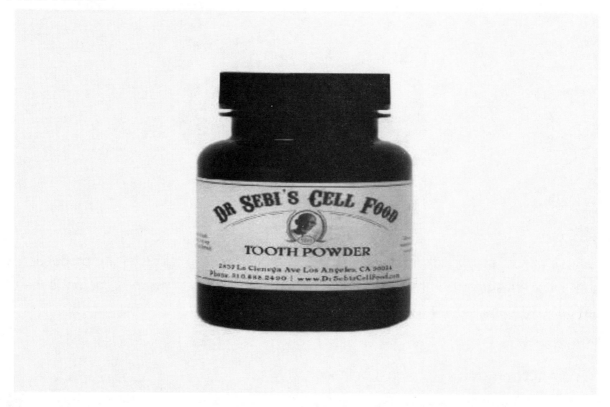

This Tooth Powder aids in the treatment of tooth decay and gum disease.

Ingredients:

- Encino
- Myrrh Gum Powder

Uterine Wash & Oil

Cleanses and replenishes the vaginal flora and fauna. Red clover (Trifolium pratense) is a natural blood purifier, expectorant, and circulatory stimulant. Red clover contains flavonoids and isoflavones, both of which create oestrogen in the body. Red clover can help with a variety of menopausal symptoms.

Ingredients:

- Arnica
- Lupulo
- Red Clover
- Sage

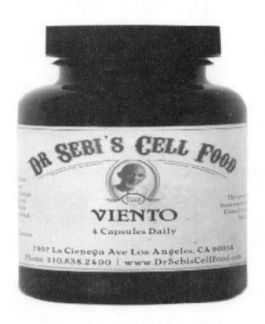

Viento

Viento is a tonic, cleanser, and rejuvenator. Chaparral (Larrea Tridentate) has been identified as an effective antioxidant. Chaparral was utilised by Native Americans to cure a variety of diseases, including respiratory problems, chickenpox, snake bites, and arthritic pain. Chapel is a fantastic cure for liver health, blood cleansing, immunological strengthening, weight reduction, and general wellbeing because to its potent antioxidant effects. It is also used to treat digestive and respiratory issues including cramping and gas.

Ingredients:

- Hombre Grande
- Bladderwrack

- Valeriana

- Chaparral

- Hierba del Sapo

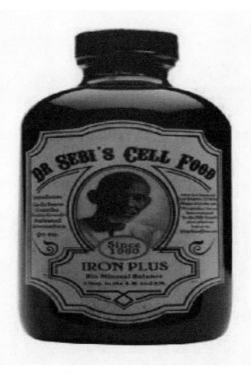

Iron Plus

Iron plus purifies the entire body. Chaparral (Larrea Tridentate) has been shown to be a potent antioxidant. Chaparral was utilised by Native Americans to cure a variety of diseases, including respiratory problems, chickenpox, snake bites, and arthritic pain. Chaparral is extremely useful for liver health, blood purification, immune boosting, weight loss, and overall wellbeing due to its potent antioxidant capabilities. It is also used to treat digestive and respiratory issues including cramping and gas.

Ingredients:

- Bugleweed

- Chaparral

- Elderberry

- Blue Vernvain

- Palo Guaco

- Hombre Grande

Dr. Sebi's Nerve/Stress Relief Herbal Tea

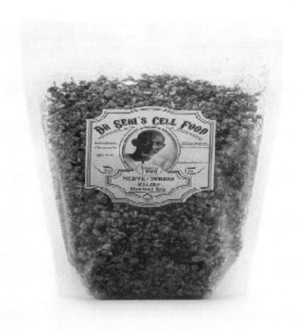

Dr. Sebi Natural Chamomile Tea supports good sleep and relaxation in a gentle manner. Chamomile serves as a moderate sedative and may boost mood, as well as soothing muscle groups and decreasing irritation. Chamomile's anti-inflammatory, antibacterial, and antioxidant properties help to alleviate irritable bowel syndrome and other gastrointestinal issues.

Use instructions: 2 cups distilled water, boiled Sebi's nerves/stress relief Soak for 10-15 minutes before drinking in the evening.

 Ingredients:

- Chamomile

Dr. Sebi's Stomach Relief Herbal Tea

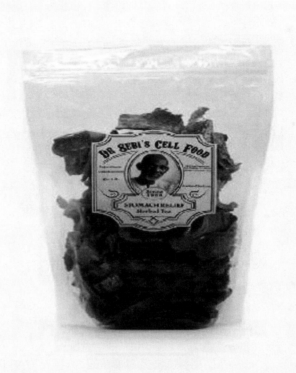

Stomach Relief by Dr. Sebi Cuachalalate (Amphipterygium astringens) tea is brewed from a famous plant used in Central America to heal most abdominal problems, including stomach cancer, stomach ulcers, and kidney sickness. Natural infusions have historically been used to relieve discomfort and suffering in the urinary system and kidneys caused by stomach ulcers, mouth illnesses, or small ulcers. Use instructions: 2 cups pure water, plus 112 tablespoons Dr. Sebi's tea 15 minutes in the oven Allow to cool before straining. It must be consumed twice day.

Ingredients:

- Cuachalalate

Dr. Sebi's Blood Pressure Balance Herbal Tea

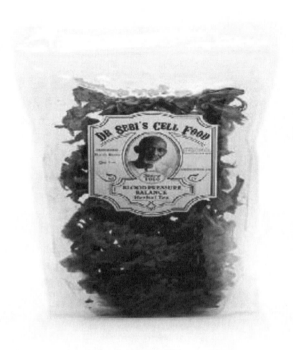

Dr. Sebi's Floor de Manita herbal tea is intended to help regulate high or low blood pressure. Mexican Handflowers (chiranthodendron) have been used for ages to treat heart disease and stomach discomfort. A higher frequency of consumption may assist to lower blood cholesterol levels and improve cardiovascular health.

Preparation:

2 cups of clean water, 2 tablespoons Dr. Sebi's Blood Pressure Balance Herbal Tea Allow it to cool and settle for approximately 15 minutes after it comes to a boil. Take it twice each day.

Ingredients:

- Flor de Manita

Dr. Sebi's Cold/Cough Herbal Tea

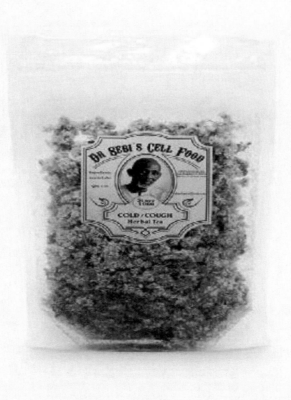

Dr. Sebi's Gordolobo herbal tea rapidly improves phlegm associated with colds or flu. Although it helps to ease coughs by somewhat reducing mucus, it can also be used to treat bronchitis, sore throat, pneumonia, fever, sore throat, and intestinal illnesses that cause diarrhoea or gastroenteritis.

Preparation:

To Dr. Sebi's, add two glasses of purified water and two teaspoons of cold / cough herbal tea. Boil for 10-15 minutes, drain, and consume twice daily.

Ingredients:

- Gordolobo

Advanced Package

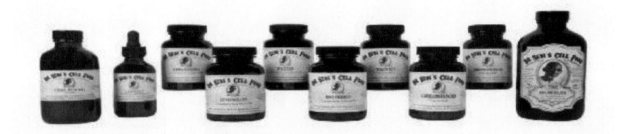

The enhanced package includes special components that help to accelerate the healing process. This package promotes rejuvenation, intercellular improvement, and quicker detoxification.

Products Included (10 products):

- Chelation 2
- Bromide Plus Capsules
- Lymphalin
- Fucus Capsules
- Lupulo
- Chelation 1
- Viento
- Iron Plus
- Green Food

- Bio Ferro Capsules

All-Inclusive Package (Male – Testo)

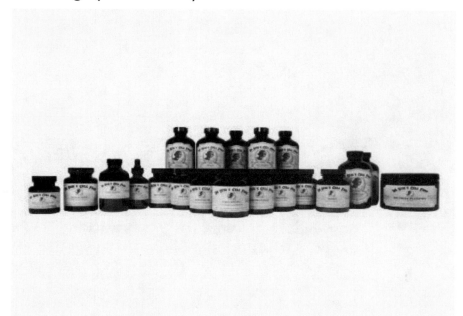

All of our clients recommend the "All Inclusive" package for males since it cleanses the entire body on a cellular level by breaking down acid, mucus, toxins, and calcifications. It rebuilds and revitalises the body, as well as the blood and immune system.

The saturation rate in this package is the highest: the higher the saturation rate, the faster and more effective the cleansing results.

Products Included (20 products):

- Fucus Capsules
- Chelation 2
- Chelation 1
- Fucus Liquid
- Bromide Plus Capsules
- Lymphalin
- L.O.V.
- Banju (2)
- Bio Ferro Tonic (2)

- Lupulo

- Bromide Plus Powder

- Green Food

- Estro

- Viento

- Iron Plus (2)

- Endocrine

- Bio Ferro Capsules

All-Inclusive Package (Female – Estro)

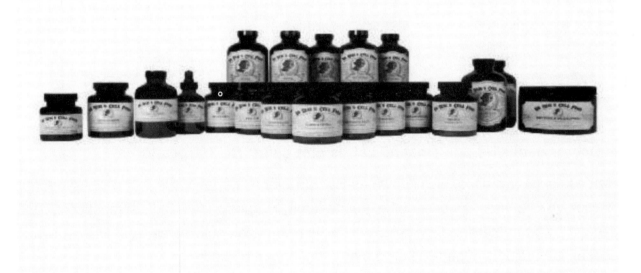

Because it cleanses the entire body on a cellular level by breaking down acid, mucus, toxins, and calcifications, the "All Inclusive" package for women is recommended for all of our clients. It rebuilds and revitalises the body, as well as the blood and immune system.

The saturation rate in this package is the highest: the higher the saturation rate, the faster and more effective the cleansing results.

Products Included (20 products):

- Chelation 1
- Lymphalin
- Fucus Capsules
- Fucus Liquid
- L.O.V.
- Chelation 2
- Lupulo
- Banju (2)
- Bromide Plus Powder
- Bio Ferro Capsules
- Viento
- Iron Plus (2)
- Endocrine
- Green Food
- Bromide Plus Capsules
- Estro

Is Doctor Sebi's Herpes Treatm? Let us first define the Herpes Virus.

Herpes simplex viruses, also known as Human Alpha Herpes Virus 1 and Human Alpha Herpes Virus 2, are members of the human family Herpesviridae and are most commonly caused by viral infections. Both HSV-1 (which produces cold sores) and HSV-2 (which causes the majority of genital herpes) are common and infectious.

Dr. Sebi's healing abilities had become a godsend to millions of people, and among those treated were some people infected with the Herpes Virus.

The health-care industry is worth billions of dollars, which is why huge pharmaceutical companies sued Dr. Sebi the instant he discovered a 1-WEEK CURE FOR HERPES (Oral and Genital). Dr. Sebi stated that a combination of Alkaline Food and home cures may be employed to build great electric components to revitalise the body.

Prior to his death, Dr. Sebi's goal was to establish an ideal society devoid of health issues and illnesses, but he redirected a lot of money to English pharmaceuticals, which may no longer help his cause. When it comes to treating HERPES (Genital/Oral), anti-retroviral tablets will cause more harm than benefit.

BOOK 6
Dr. Sebi Treatment and Cures PART II

How to Cure Cancer, Diabetes, Lupus, Herpes, HIV, Hair Loss, and Other Diseases Using Dr. Sebi's Alkaline Diet

Dr. Sebi's Approach to Reversing Diabetes

Before we go into Dr. Sebi's strategy, let's define diabetes.

Diabetes is a condition that causes a rise in your blood sugar level, often known as blood sugar. Blood sugar is your major source of energy, and it is obtained from the meals you consume. Insulin, a hormone produced by the pancreas, facilitates the entry of glucose into your cells to give energy.

Sometimes your body does not produce enough – or any – insulin, or it may not utilise insulin effectively. The glucose is subsequently stored in your blood and does not reach your cells. When you have too much glucose in your blood, it might create health complications. Although the medical community thinks that diabetes cannot be cured, there are actions you may take to control diabetes and stay healthy. Dr. Sebi, a famous herbalist, however, has a remedy that has lasted the test of time.

According to Dr. Sebi, having a bio-mineral balance is the foundation for cleansing the body of all ailments, including diabetes. Many people have reported being called by Dr. Sebi to be cared for and cured. Dr. Sebi's therapy for type 2 diabetes is straightforward: follow his nutritional advice, eliminate bad cells, and oxygenate the healthy cells.

Dr. Sebi's Herbs for Diabetes

Dr. Sebi has recommended the following herbs for use in reversing and curing diabetes:

- Dandelion
- Bitter Melon / Cerasee
- Bilberry / Blueberry Leaves
- Guinea Hen Basil
- RootFig LeavesGuaco
- Herb Seville /Sour Orange

- Weed Ginger
- Root Huereque / Wereke Holy
- Herb Hoodia
- Seeds Nopal
- Leaves Milk
- Thistle
- Gordonii Mango
- Herb Seville /Sour Orange
- Okra
- Prodigiosa
- Raspberry
- Leaves Sage
- Cactus

Dr. Sebi's Herbal Formula for Diabetes

- Bromide Plus
- Endocrine Formula

Remedies and Cures For Lupus

Lupus, also known as systemic lupus erythematosus, is an auto-immune disease in which your immune system fights against your own organs and tissues as well as external intruders. Lupus is a chronic disease that causes inflammation of your joints, skin, and other organs. Although there is no cure for lupus, the long-term impacts and symptoms of the disease can be managed better by early identification and therapy.

People with lupus can expect to live an ordinary life if they receive sufficient care. The Lupus Foundation of America claims this. Some of these drugs and therapies will be evaluated in the near future. Before we get there, let's look at some of the most prevalent lupus symptoms. This includes symptoms such as chest discomfort, swollen lymph nodes, and painful and swollen joints. There is also fever, hair loss, and mouth ulcers.

Herbs Used for The Treatment of Lupus

Tumeric

Tumeric lowers lupus inflammation. Curcumin is one of the active components in Lupus. Curcumin is effective in the treatment of autoimmune diseases such as lupus. Tumeric can be added to a meal or, better yet, consumed as a drink. Add a teaspoon to your milk, heat it, and drink. You may also consume it with honey to improve the flavour. Before you begin taking Turmeric, consult with your doctor. Turmeric cannot be taken with honey if you have gallbladder problems. It is harmful to them.

Ginger

Ginger, with its anti-oxidant and anti-inflammatory qualities, aids in the reduction of pain and swelling. Ginger can be ingested in the form of juice and tea, or it can be added to food. Its curative therapy is necessary for a variety of health issues.

Apple Cider Vinegar

A lupus patient is lacking in hydrochloric acid. According to a medical professional. Apple cider vinegar stimulates the body's synthesis of hydrochloric acid. It increased nutrition absorption and aided in detoxifying. This alone is reason enough to make an apple cider vinegar drink. Take a cup of warm water, add a teaspoon of apple cider vinegar, and half a lemon juice, and drink it 20 minutes before your meal. Do it three times a day.

Coconut Oil

Coconut oil provides a plethora of health advantages, including improved digestion; it also regulates blood sugar and cholesterol levels in the body. Coconut oil can help you balance out the negative effects of your immune system on your body. Coconut oil may be used to prepare your meals as well as to consume drinks.

Tulsi Or Holy Basil

Holy Basil is utilised to prevent flare-ups and to control your stress level. Lupus flare-ups are caused by a high amount of stress on your immune system. Anti-inflammatory and anti-oxidant qualities of holy basil aid to reduce tiredness, enhance organ function, and provide a sense of well-being. Basil may be taken by creating a herbal tea out of it and drinking it three times a day. You may also eat the basil leaves on a daily basis.

Epsom Salt

Epsom Salt aids in the absorption of magnesium and the removal of toxins from the body. It also aids in the reduction of joint discomfort and inflammation. The use of an Epsom salt bath can help with fatigue, which is one of the symptoms of lupus. To make an Epsom salt bath, add a cup of Epsom salt to your bathwater and thoroughly mix it in. Then immerse yourself in it for 20 to 30 minutes to allow your body to absorb it properly. Patients with kidney disease and diabetics are not eligible.

Flaxseeds

Flaxseed contains a high concentration of omega-3 fatty acids. This helps lupus sufferers decrease inflammation and enhance renal function. As a lupus patient, take 30 grammes of flaxseeds each day to overcome renal or kidney failure.

Green Tea

According to the findings of the study, green tea extracts supplied to a lupus patient over a 12-week period assist treat lupus symptoms and flare-ups.

Medication Use for The Treatment Of Lupus

Medicine is mostly used to treat lupus and can be used alone or in combination. This is depends on your specific situation. However, the actions of various medications varies.

Their common feature is that they assist minimise edoema in your body. Lupus is treated using the medications listed below.

NSAID

Ibuprofen, aspirin, indomethacin, and Naprosyn are medications used to treat edoema, discomfort, and stiffness. These medications are effective in controlling lupus symptoms.

Antimalarial drugs.

Researchers discovered that medications used to treat malaria, such as hydroxychloroquine, can also be used to treat lupus flares. These antimalarial medications aid in the reduction of joint swelling and skin rashes. It can be used alone to treat mild to severe lupus. For severe instances involving the kidneys and other organs, hydroxychloroquine (Plaquenil) should be administered in conjunction with other medications.

According to a Harvard Medical School associate professor of medicine, antimalaria medications have become a daily multivitamin for persons with mild to moderate lupus. Despite the modest side effects, these medications can help avoid issues, so enhancing your health in the long run.

Benlysta

This medication is an antibody that not only identifies but also inhibits protein in the immune system. The protein contributes to the immune system's attack on your body's cells. Benlysta, commonly known as Belimumab, is the most recent lupus medication to be authorised in 2011. It's used to treat lupus. To be successful, this treatment must be taken in conjunction with other lupus medications. Some lupus patients benefit from this medication because it lessens the amount of steroids they must take. This can have unpleasant adverse effects on them; it does nothing for the other half of the lupus population. Fever, nausea, and diarrhoea are some of the negative effects of Benlysta usage.

Cortiscosteroids

Oral steroids such as Prednisolone and Prednisone can help those suffering from a severe lupus flare that damages their organs. A large dose of it can aid the patient by reducing their symptoms. The use of steroids does have negative effects, such as mood changes, sadness, and weight gain. Steroid use, if not well controlled, can lead to an increased risk of osteoporosis in the long run. Weight-related diseases such as high blood pressure and diabetes are not excluded.

According to an associate professor of medicine at Harvard Medical School, the fundamental goal of using steroids is to get the person on the lowest feasible dose required to treat symptoms. Your rheumatologist should gradually lower the dosage as you improve.

At the same time, some patients may discontinue their use. Others would most likely require long-term therapy as long as they are on low-dose steroids. There is also encouraging news for anyone suffering from lupus-related skin rashes. Steroids are now available in a tropical therapy to aid with rashes.

Immunosuppressive drugs

Immune suppressive medicines are often prescribed for persons with severe lupus and when corticosteroids have failed or are not an option. Immunosuppressive medications help the patient by alleviating symptoms. This is accomplished by suppressing your immune system. Lupus is caused by an overactive immune system.

Immunosuppressive medications are not without negative effects. Taking this medication makes you fully vulnerable to infection. As a result, anytime you observe symptoms of disease or infection, you should seek medical assistance.

Experimental medication

These novel lupus treatments are intended to target specific immune cells. Research and testing are underway. If you are interested, speak with your doctor about participating in a clinical study.

Other medication

These medications include statins, diuretics, and anticoagulants, as well as blood pressure medications, antibiotics, stimulants, and others. Lupus affects each individual differently, depending on their symptoms. As a result, the above-mentioned drugs are in great demand.

The trick is to discover the perfect mix, since no one combination is useful to people with lupus, so keep this in mind and allow your rheumatologist time to find you the right combination.

Fitzgerald claims that "A medicine may be effective in some persons but not in others. Unfortunately, we have no way of knowing who will profit and who will not."

Additional Lupus Treatments

Aside from medication, other lupus therapies include:

Transplants and surgery

This is an example of lupus affecting the organs, namely the kidneys. This causes kidney failure and need a transplant to preserve their life.

Experimental treatments

Scientists are constantly researching alternative treatments for lupus all around the world. A stem cell transplant is one of them. Only a severe case of lupus that has not responded to previous medications can be evaluated for an experimental therapy.

Complementary medicine

There is evidence that supplements such as fish oil and DHEA may be beneficial to lupus sufferers. Before beginning a supplement regimen, consult with your rheumatologist. It might either interact with the lupus or aggravate it, like a two-edged sword.

Lifestyle Change

Lupus cannot be fought solely by medical staff. You, as an individual, have a role to play in how you conduct your life. What exactly do I mean?

The foods you eat matters.

There is currently no food plan available for controlling lupus symptoms. You may help yourself by avoiding junk and acidic meals and eating more alkaline-based foods, such as fruits and vegetables. You can see your doctor for meal advice that can considerably enhance your health. Consider the following scenario: you have a kidney condition. Your doctor would most likely advise you to eat low-salt foods. Assume you were losing bone mass. Your doctor may advise you to consume calcium and vitamin D-rich foods. So, strive for a healthier diet.

Exercise regularly.

Exercise can reduce a person's risk of heart disease if they have lupus. It has the ability to increase your energy, sharpen your intellect, and greatly enhance your mood.

Stress is a killer, so reduce it

Reduce your stress levels by practising yoga, meditation, breathing techniques, and biofeedback. Another method for dealing with stress is cognitive-behavioral therapy.

Learn to rest

You must allow your body to restore itself. Find time to relax during the day, in between your obligations. Individuals with lupus also need 8 to 10 hours of sleep every night.

Working with doctors

You must have a handful of these medical people in your medical portfolio. Depending on your symptoms, a rheumatologist, a general practitioner, and other lupus experts may be consulted. Because lupus is so unpredictable, frequent check-ups are essential. A excellent therapy now may not be so nice tomorrow. These lupus symptoms are bound to change over time. Lupus fears might be an avenue as long as you obtain the care you need when you need it.

"Those diagnosed with lupus should be positive about therapy," Bermas believes. It may take some time and trial and error to find the proper therapy. The odds of discovering a solution to your problem are thus in your favour if you persevere.

Coping with lupus medication side effects

People should not be concerned about the potential negative effects of lupus. While the adverse effects of lupus medications are real and serious, and some are even unusual, the vast majority of them are manageable.

Fitzgerald is certain that "People need to understand that we know what side effects to watch for when they take these meds. If they occur, we modify the prescription, and the problem generally resolves itself."

When you discuss your concerns with your rheumatologist, he or she will be in a better position to assist you balance the potential hazards as well as the potential advantages of your lupus medication.

How to Prevent and Treat Hair Loss

Hair loss is a global issue, and about one-third of the world's population is affected by it. As you can see, it's a typical occurrence, so you shouldn't be concerned about a few stray hairs. Medication, mineral deficiency, nutrition, stress, or heredity can all cause hair loss. Putting on a hat or cap might be attributed to hair loss. This chapter provides helpful hair loss prevention strategies, some of which are detailed below.

Shampoo your hair regularly.

One method of preventing hair loss is to keep the scalp clean by washing your hair on a regular and thorough basis. This procedure reduces the danger of dandruff and infection, which can lead to hair breakage or loss.

Vitamins

Scientists believe that vitamins A, B, C, D, zinc, iron, and selenium are critical to the growth and retention of your hair, particularly with cell turnover. So you can see that vitamins are important not only for your health, but also for your hair. Vitamin A is required for the development of healthy sebum in the scalp, which keeps your scalp healthy and allows it to maintain more hair. Consume vitamin A-rich foods such as spinach, sweet pepper, sweet potato, and so on.

Vitamin B is required for the preservation of healthy hair hues. At the same time, Vitamin E promotes blood circulation around the scalp, resulting in healthy hair follicles.

Protein

A 2017 research (reliable source) found that the majority of 100 patients suffering from hair loss were nutritionally insufficient, particularly in amino acids, which are a building block of protein. At the same time, researchers believe that further study is needed to confirm the aforementioned findings (Trusted source). Because hair follicles are made up of a protein called keratin, a diet high in protein such as fish, lean meat, beans, nuts, eggs, chicken, turkey, and low-fat dairy products helps to prevent hair loss.

Massage aromatic oils onto your scalp.

To keep the hair follicles alive, combine lavender with almond or sesame oil and massage the scalp for a few minutes.

Brushing damp hair should be avoided.

This is the point at which your hair is at its weakest. Brushing it or combing it with a wide-toothed comb will only result in further hair loss. In the same vein, combing your hair regularly harms it, and if you must untangle it, run your fingers through it rather than using a comb or brush.

Diet of the Mediterranean

The Mediterranean diet consists of fresh herbs and raw vegetables. It aids in the prevention of hair loss by lowering the risk of androgenic alopecia (male or female pattern baldness) or delaying its beginning. According to a research published in the Archive of Dermatologist Research in 2017.

Ginseng

Ginseng contains phytochemicals that encourage the development of hair on the scalp. To receive the proper dose of ginseng pills, consult with your doctor. Better still, go for tropical remedies including ginseng components.

Garlic juice, onion juice, or ginger juice

Regularly rub one of these into your scalp and leave it on for one week to see a visible difference in your hair.

Apply green tea to your hair.

Allow two bags of green tea to cool before applying to your hair and rinsing after an hour. If you do this on a regular basis for a week to ten days, you will see a major difference in your hair. According to research, putting green tea on your hair can help prevent hair loss.

De-stress There is medical data that suggests a link between hair loss and stress. De-stress yourself by practising yoga, meditation, or other stress-relieving activities. This procedure has also resulted in the restoration of your body's hormonal equilibrium.

Continuous heating and drying of your hair

Constant drying and heating of your hair makes it delicate, which leads to hair loss. The reason behind this is because the heating and drying processes weaken the protein in the hair.

Maintain hydration.

Drink at least 4 to 8 glasses of water every day to keep hydrated, since your hair shaft is around one-quarter water.

Identify what is harmful to your hair.

Allow your hair to dry naturally, as opposed to drying it mechanically. Do not massage your hair with a dry cloth. One method to maintain your hair healthy is to know what works for it.

Avoid smoking and limit your alcohol consumption.

Smoking and drinking reduce hair development by decreasing the quantity of blood that passes into the scalp. So, if you want to see an increase in hair growth, stop consuming both.

Physical exercises

Engaging in physical activities such as walking, riding, or swimming for 30 minutes every day helps to minimise hair loss, as well as reduce stress and balance your hormones.

Keep your head sweat-free.

People with oily hair get dandruff throughout the summer as a consequence of perspiration, which causes a high incidence of hair loss. To prevent dandruff, keep your hair cool by using shampoo containing neem and aloe-vera.

People who work a lot while wearing a helmet, notably myself, sweat a lot during the summer, weakening the hair and causing hair loss.

In this circumstance, wearing a terrycloth headband, scarf, or bandana over your hair will help reduce hair loss.

Your Well-Being

Make sure you take adequate care of your health. Consult your doctor if you have a high temperature, a persistent sickness, or an infection and want to have better, healthier hair.

Take note of your medicines.

Hair loss can occur as a result of drug side effects. If you see your hair coming out while taking medication, consult your doctor and request a prescription adjustment.

Chemicals should be avoided.

When your hair is falling out, do not dye it. Also, avoid using permanent hair dye, which contains harsh chemicals that might harm your hair.

Make an appointment with your doctor on a regular basis.

Consult your doctor if you have any underlying illnesses, or a dermatologist if you have any skin disorders, as they might create changes in your hormonal balance, causing your hair to fall out.

Biotin (Vitamin H)

If you have a hair loss problem, biotin-rich diet is your best friend. Biotin is a vitamin B complex that assists our bodies in converting food into energy. So eating biotin-rich foods like eggs, sweet potatoes, oats, and onions, as well as taking biotin pills, will help slow down hair loss.

Olive Oil

Dr. Sebi's diet includes olive oil, which may be used to nourish hair, protecting it from dryness and breakage and slowing down hereditary hair loss. A couple of teaspoons of it applied to your hair for thirty minutes before washing will do the trick.

Coconut Oil

Because of the lauric acid included in coconut oil, it helps bind the protein in hair, keeping it from splitting at the root and strand, according to a reliable source.

According to a 2018 research, coconut oil might help to prevent hair damage caused by grooming or exposure to UV radiation. Also, rubbing coconut oil into your scalp improves blood circulation, which helps to strengthen your hair.

What Causes Hair Loss?

Everything in life follows a circle. The same is true for your hair as it goes through its growing, resting, and shedding cycle. Losing 100 hair follicles every day is normal, but if you notice sudden hair loss in spots or overall thinning, please consult your doctor, as there may be a health issue that needs to be addressed. Hair loss occurs in stages. Some hair loss is transient and may be helped by a change in food, therapy, or even lifestyle. At the same time, another sort of shedding might be permanent, necessitating the assistance of a medical professional to shed further light on the issue.

Hereditary hair loss begins around the age of 40 for males and around the age of 70 for women, and approximately half of the population is predicted to have hair loss owing to a disorder known as androgenic alopecia (male/female pattern baldness).

Cancer radiation therapy, the way you treated your hair over time, such as cornrows or a ponytail, hormonal changes from a thyroid problem, menopause, childbirth, or pregnancy, a medical condition such as trichotillomania (hair-pulling disorder), or a scalp infection.

Finally, if you notice sudden hair loss, it is essential to schedule an appointment with your doctor because there may be some difficulties that you are unaware of. Also, keep in mind that certain hair treatments require patience because it may take longer to see a substantial difference if you have hair damage or loss.

How to Get Cancer Treatment Naturally (Food And Herbs For Body Cleansing)

There are several herbs that are indicated for cancer prevention, and these plants are supported by research. Some plants having anticancer effects are listed below.

Garlic (Allium sativum) (Allium sativum)

Sulphur, flavonoids, selenium, and arginine are all found in garlic. Garlic belongs to the onion family Alliaceae, and the bioactive molecule present in garlic is generated from allicin when cut up. The European Prospective Investigation into Cancer and Nutrition (EPIC) has discovered a favourable correlation between ingesting garlic or onions and the influence it has on cancer risk in an ongoing global investigation across ten nations.

Even research from France, China, and the United States have all corroborated EPIC's conclusion that garlic intake lowers the risk of cancer. Because of its anti-bacterial qualities, garlic has the capacity to prevent the activation and production of cancer-causing chemicals. The World Health Organization recommends one garlic bulb or 2 to 5 grammes of garlic each day for any adult who is serious about battling cancer.

Ginger (Zingiber officinale) (Zingiber officinale)

Ginger is a member of the Zingiberaceae family and has been used medicinally for for 2,000 years. Ginger's anti-inflammatory and antioxidant capabilities have been proven in an experimental model to be particularly effective in preventing cancer progression. Ginger has been shown in studies to prevent cancer, such as one conducted at Michigan University, where ginger induced ovarian cancer cells to die. Not to mention the study published in Cancer Prevention Research, which found that consuming ginger reduced colon inflammation significantly.

While science is doing everything it can to battle cancer, you, as a person, have a role to play in preventing cancer from knocking on your door. Consume foods that are high in fruits and vegetables while limiting your intake of foods that are acidic in nature. This is how you can protect yourself, your family, and remain healthy.

Amla

According to Ayurveda, a philosophy that originated in India more than 5,000 years ago, amla is a superfood known as the rejuvenation king because it is one of the highest sources of Vitamin C. Gallic acid, quercetin, tannins, flavonoids, pectin, and numerous polyphenolic substances are found in it. The ancient usage of amla has been confirmed once again to be correct by scientific study conducted over three decades, and laboratory trials employing amla extracts have been successful against malignant cells without injuring the individual using it.

Tumeric

Tumeric is one of the most investigated herbs for its anti-cancer effects, as well as anti-inflammatory, antibacterial, anti-oxidant, and analgesic characteristics. Turmeric's major component is curcumin. It contains strong antioxidant qualities that help to prevent the formation of malignant cells in the body. According to 2,000 published research articles, curcumin can kill malignant cells without damaging healthy ones.

Ashwagandha

Researchers found the anti-cancer benefit of Indian ginseng over 40 years ago when they extracted the crystalline steroidal ingredient (withaferin A) from this plant. In Ayurveda, ashwagandha is used to assist the body cope with stress. Cancerous cells were discovered to be killed by extracts extracted from the Ashwagandha leaf.

Basil (Ocimum basilicum)

Basil is a culinary herb well recognised for its medicinal properties. Tulsi is the name given to it in India because it is indigenous to the country. Not only that, but it may also be found in Iran and other tropical Asian countries.

Basil is now accessible all over the world. Basil's antiviral, antibacterial, antimutagenic, antitumorigenic, and antioxidant effects were derived from numerous components, including estragole, eugenol, linalool, and 1,8-cineole.

According to study, basil is used to combat stress and boost immunity since it also has analgesic, anti-diabetic, anti-stress, and anti-inflammatory qualities. According to research, the phytochemicals found in basil prevent chemically generated lung, liver, oral, and skin cancers by modifying gene expression, enhancing antioxidant activity, and preventing cancer from spreading to other organs.

Dr. Sebi's Herpes Cure

Herpes is a viral ailment caused by the herpes simplex virus. There is no cure. However, there are medicines available to assist herpes patients manage their symptoms.

Herpes comes in two varieties: herpes simplex virus 1 (HSV-1) and herpes simplex virus 2 (HSV-2) (HSV-2). Despite the fact that both cause genital herpes, only HSV-1 causes oral herpes.

Herpes symptoms include sores on the skin, mouth, genitals, and anal region. Dr. Sebi's herpes therapies are included below to assist you control your symptoms.

Honey

According to a 2019 study, the use of Kanuka honey in the form of antiviral lotions is beneficial in treating oral herpes. According to the study, it took 9 days with honey and 8 days with antiviral cream to treat the sores. At the same time, without therapy, oral herpes can cure in 1-2 weeks. It is unclear whether the ability to cure is limited to Kanuka honey or all honey in general.

Vitamins

Vitamins have a critical role in protecting the body from the herpes virus and its effects.

A high vitamin D level can assist enhance a section of your immune system, protecting your body from this infection. A lack of vitamin D, on the other hand, makes your system an accessible target for the herpes virus.

The antioxidative characteristics of vitamin E can help minimise the stress exerted on your immune system by herpes, lowering the likelihood of infection. According to reports, vitamin E is being used in clinical studies to treat herpes. Taking supplements or other dietary changes can help increase the amount of these vitamins in your body. Sunlight is another way to increase your vitamin D level in your body.

Garlic

Garlic has many therapeutic effects in general, and its medical usage in addressing most disorders dates back several centuries, particularly for both forms of herpes. It is typically boiled and consumed as tea, taken in capsule form, or eaten fresh. Allicin, a chemical found in garlic, has been shown to have both preventative and therapeutic effects on the herpes simplex virus; however, there is no conclusive proof as of yet.

Gels

If you have genital herpes, you may readily purchase gels designed to alleviate the discomfort associated with urinating. However, it has been shown that just putting petroleum jelly to the afflicted region alleviates the agony. It is critical to wash both hands prior to and after application.

Dietary changes

Diet has always had a significant influence in either enhancing or inhibiting an individual's immune system and overall health.

For decades, pomegranate has been used as an excellent home treatment for infections. This fruit is abundant in zinc, which helps to decrease herpes infections.

Increasing lysine diet while avoiding arginine has been shown to be effective in the prevention and treatment of herpes infection. Lysine sources include cheese and pork, whereas Arginine sources include soy protein, salmon, walnuts, and peanuts.

Reduced use of red wine, caffeine, and heavy smoking has been shown to help with herpes infection control.

It is also useful in the prevention and management of HSV to recognise and avoid dietary items that cause allergies.

Supplements

According to previous research, zinc, lysine, lemon balm, adenosine monophosphate, vitamin E, and vitamin C can all help to manage herpes symptoms.

Taking lysine supplements, according to the International Council on Amino Acid Science, can help reduce cold sore breakouts.

According to researchers in a 2017 analysis, a minimum of 1 gramme of lysine for one day, along with a low arginine diet, can assist patients deal with their symptoms. To avoid bad side effects, always contact with your doctor before using supplements, since there is a significant risk that they will mix with other drugs, resulting in an unanticipated unpleasant side effect.

Oil

HSV-1 can be reduced by using oil-like wormwood, hinoki cypress, rosemary, garden thyme, eucalyptus caesia, Tripterygium hypoglaucum, basil, and cinnamon.

Apart than taking them orally, these oils may be combined in your bathwater or used in a diffuser to directly affect the HSV regions.

It should be noted that applying them straight to the skin without diluting them may result in negative effects, thus dilute them with carrier oils such as almond and olive oil.

Although there is no confirmed proof that oil can help with herpes symptoms, scientific research are underway to see if organic oils like jojoba oil and sesame oil have the ability to treat herpes symptoms.

Prevention And Recovering From Herpes

Herpes is, as previously said, an infectious virus with no treatment. Simultaneously, HIV is a Human Immune Virus that has no cure and may be caught when people participate in a high-risk behaviour, such as unprotected intercourse with an infected person, whether intentionally or unknowingly. So, what are the procedures to follow to either recover if you've already been affected or, better yet, prevent becoming infected by this virus?

It is reasonable to conclude that persons with herpes may be at an elevated risk of contracting HIV since the same factors that put them at risk for one infection, such as not using condoms or having anonymous or many partners, may also put them at risk for another, in this case HIV. Because herpes and HIV are related, it is clear that when someone contracts herpes, he or she got it from someone who was at risk of contracting both herpes and HIV.

It has been demonstrated that persons with herpes can increase the risk of HIV transmission.

You are indulging in anal, oral, or vaginal intercourse without wearing a condom, which might raise your risk of Herpes and HIV.

Having several partners

Having intercourse while under the influence of alcohol or drugs increases your risk.

Having sex partners who are not identified.

So, can treating herpes protect against HIV?

Not quite correct. Though treating herpes should reduce the risk of HIV significantly, studies have shown that it does not. Herpes therapy reduces problems and even transmission to our loved ones, but it does not halt the spread of HIV.

Use a condom and dental dam for every act of anal, vaginal, or oral intercourse from start to end. Stick to one partner, and if you must have a new partner, speak honestly between yourselves about having a test to check whether you are infected prior to having sex.

Don't participate in any sexual activity when high on drugs or alcohol; instead, have an honest chat with yourself and take a test. Many people prefer not to know what is going on in their bodies, but for the benefit of you and your loved ones, this is not the ideal way to live.

Consult your doctor about pre-exposure prophylaxis (PREP) and post-exposure prophylaxis (PEP). Determine which choice is best for you and your partner to avoid HIV infection.

We now know that people who have herpes are twice as likely as people who do not have herpes to obtain HIV. People who are infected with both are more likely to transmit them on to others, therefore it is in your best interest to avoid dangerous behaviour. Assist in the protection of yourself and your family.

BOOK 7
DR. SEBI APPROVED
HERBS

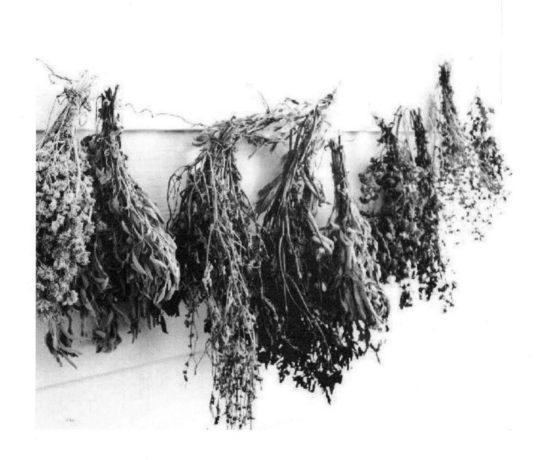

The Ultimate Guide to Naturally Detox Your Body with Dr. Sebi Herbs

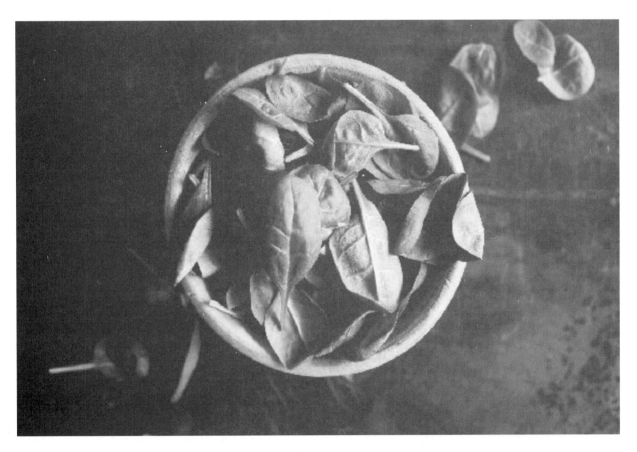

The drive for a balanced and healthy lifestyle in our culture today has unlocked the treasure trove of age-old health practices like yoga, Ayurveda, and the usage of herbs to enhance our health. Even though these techniques occasionally lack scientific support or endorsement, they are quite effective at restoring people's health. Although this has lessened the need for modern medicine, the overall objective of promoting health is still achieved; therefore, it makes little difference whether you use a pill or a herbal remedy.

Although plants were used thousands of years ago in ancient Egypt, Greece, and China, Dr. Sebi discovered a way to open up their world. This information delves into Dr. Sebi's herbal notebook, which he identified as a reliable source of treatments for several ailments. Dr. Sebi's main objective is to keep patients healthy rather than treat their illnesses. He discovered that if our bodies are kept in a certain state, it will often be difficult to get sick; therefore, he developed his alkaline diet.

These alkaline diets are ideal for body detoxification or eliminating toxic toxins from the body. These diets include all food groups and are largely vegan. Still, our attention is on herbs because they can support our bodies' natural functions. Due to the enormous amount of poisonous compounds we ingest daily, detoxing your body is essential for everyone. However, knowing what to do and avoid will have the same effect.

The Importance of Detoxing and Revitalizing Your Body

The human body always tries to eliminate harmful compounds and toxins from various organs. Unhealthy foods, alcohol, narcotics, coffee, stress, and other factors weaken the human body over time. Due to the rise in industrial waste, these environmental poisons are everywhere.

Several external variables always place our body's system in an unhealthy state, despite the deliberate effort we might make to maintain a good diet or lifestyle. The next step is for our body to eliminate things that can prohibit us from having excellent health.

Toxins force our vital organs to work harder than they would otherwise, which eventually wears them out, reduces their effectiveness, and increases the risk of sickness.

Making time to cleanse the body's organs and lessen the stress these organs experience will go a long way toward preventing further illness. This method produces advantages that are seen right away, such as improved digestion, more energy, and clearer skin. What is detoxification, therefore, given this?

Detoxification, often known as detox, is the process of removing toxic, poisonous, or damaging chemicals from the body through physical or medical means. The liver is primarily responsible for this process. It can be understood as the period of withdrawal that permits the body to return to homeostasis following a protracted period of additional consumption. In medicine, removing the harmful intake and using antidotes can speed up detoxification. Methods like chelation therapy and dialysis can only be used in a select few situations.

Where Do Toxins Come From?

In the past, we produced our food using only natural methods, including pest control, composite manure, and fertilizers. That era is quickly passing away as we increasingly rely on refined, packaged meals with lots of preservatives and meat, fish, and milk from industrial farms.

The main issue is the use of pesticides, synthetic fertilizers, and increased hormones in modern farming. Additionally, numerous pesticides and herbicides are permitted when food is genetically modified (GMO). We now eat more poisons due to the widespread use of genetically engineered foods and products.

These toxins can have disastrous effects when mixed with airborne pollutants like carbon monoxide from car exhaust pipes, pollution from factories, agricultural wastes, and pollutants dumped in our waterways. Additionally, it can be found in residues of the chemicals used to purify our drinking water, such as chlorine.

Types of Detoxification

Alcohol Detoxification: Alcohol detoxification is the process of purging and restoring your body's system to its healthy state after it has been affected by an excessive amount of alcohol. GABA neurotransmitter receptors are devalued by alcohol addiction, and abruptly quitting a long-term alcohol habit without competent medical support can result in serious and even fatal health issues. Alcohol detox is not a part of treating alcoholism; instead, alternative therapies should be employed to break the addiction that alcohol consumption has created.

Drug Detoxification: Drug detoxification is a technique physicians use to lessen withdrawal symptoms while assisting a drug user in adjusting to life without drugs. The goal of drug detoxification is not to treat addiction but rather to represent the first steps in long-term treatment. Detoxification can be carried out without the use of pharmaceuticals or may do so in conjunction with medication. Instead of taking place in a hospital, drug detoxification and treatment frequently occur in community programs that span several months. Drug detoxification shifts the focus of treatment placement. Still, some detox facilities offer therapy to mitigate the physical withdrawal symptoms from alcohol and other drugs; these additions include therapy and counseling during detox to help with the effect of withdrawal.

It is time to regain your health as soon as you become aware of a balancing issue. However, it is always challenging when the consequences of prolonged excess weigh heavily on you; in this situation, a detox might be helpful as a sufficient cure. People become drowsy owing to a lack of sleep, poor energy levels, and inactivity in daily tasks. You will undoubtedly wish to do some cleansing procedures on your body and mind and refresh your entire system.

Here are some of the most effective methods for doing so:

According to Mary McGuire, owner of the Rosenberg American Yogini in New York, "It's excellent to do the same with your body and detoxify twice a year when the seasons change, just like you clean your home in the spring and winter."

If you can cleanse yourself, it shows you have some commitment and discipline. Previous detoxers allegedly vouch for how it improved their energy and mental clarity and made their complexion gleam. If you are new to detoxing, going on a retreat for a few days and experiencing a lifestyle radically different from their regular dietary poisons can yield the finest benefits. You should avoid meat and focus on fresh, organic fruit and vegetable juice, which will be much easier to maintain when you are away from home. Other recommended foods include grains, fish, and fiber.

In addition to restoring healthy energy, stress-free sleep, and overall well-being, a three- to five-day retreat can help some people lose up to 20 pounds in two weeks and up to 5-7 pounds in a week. People feel hunger pangs, desires, and sickness after the first three days of tasking discipline since low blood sugar no longer exists.

Is Your Body in Need of a Detox?

1. Observe the warning indicators listed below;

2. Stress makes you fast and weary.

3. You experience ongoing headaches and a loss of mental clarity.

4. You occasionally get skin blemishes and outbreaks, and your complexion is dull.

5. You are frequently taking medication and prone to getting colds, bugs, the flu, and some viruses.

6. You occasionally have issues, such as painful digestion.

7. You frequently consume less healthful things like iced meat, dairy, refined meals, refined sugar, and fried foods.

8. You frequently consume coffee, drugs, alcohol, cigarettes, etc.

9. You often encounter environmental contaminants such as household chemicals, carbon emissions, pesticides, and herbicides.

10. Due to your excess body weight, you feel heavy.

11. You struggle with depression regularly because of erratic emotions, a lack of

available energy, and a general lack of excitement for life.

12. No matter how frequently you brush your teeth or bathe, you occasionally encounter bad breath and body odor.

How to Naturally Detox Your Body?

Although we all cleanse for different reasons, the main goal of detoxification is to get rid of toxins from the body. The liver, which is considered the blood's filter by eliminating toxins from the body system, is the primary organ in the body in charge of detoxification.

Toxin buildup within the body might prevent the liver from operating at its best. It will help the liver and other important organs to purify the blood and other organs to work efficiently when you incorporate detoxification practices into your lifestyle.

Because they are in the cleaning supplies, cosmetics, food, water we use for drinking and bathing, and the air we breathe, toxins are constantly bombarding us (mostly those in sealed cans).

The toxic burden on our system rises along with our level of mental stress. Once there has been a buildup, you can eventually show signs and symptoms of a widespread, severe form of inflammation in the body, which is the root cause of many chronic illnesses.

Although our bodies are indeed capable of fighting these poisons, it is also known that sometimes they overwhelm our bodies' natural capacity for healing, necessitating the need for a process like a detox process to help our bodies recover. The body can be improved in several ways, including through dieting management and other self-care practices.

Body Detox Benefits

Applying detox in a healthy method can be a great strategy to improve the condition of your body. This may assist in treating newly discovered symptoms and reduce the likelihood that the poisons may further harm you. Here are a few beneficial post-detox changes you might encounter.

Enhanced Energy

By taking detoxifying nutrients, you may remove pollutants and waste from your body system. This improves digestion, makes you feel lighter and more energized, and reduces inflammation.

Lessening of Stress

When a physical detox takes place, stress triggers like deep sleep, refined carbohydrates, and coffee are simultaneously being eliminated from the body. Additionally, intentional self-care helps ease mental stress, and detoxes can assist the body get rid of pollutants and congestion.

Loss of weight

You are typically relieved of the reliance and cravings related to processed meals and added sugar, which frequently causes weight gain. You can lose weight by managing your stress levels and making deliberate diet and portion choices.

Gut happier

The liver's capacity for cleansing can be increased by detoxification. We may experience gas, bloating, and constipation if the liver is not functioning correctly.

How to Detox Your Body?

Celebrities are well renowned for their body detoxes, which typically include (leech therapy, fasting, or colonic irrigation). However, due to its complexity, not every strategy focused on preventing the accumulation of contaminants has been successful.

The experts-recommended techniques for reducing toxins in the body are listed below. You should also be aware that a few detoxification techniques have not received adequate scrutiny. Since their exact results are therefore unknown, it is advisable to get a doctor's recommendation before beginning any detoxification. Specific detox methods or levels of detox may be prohibited for some people, such as nursing mothers, pregnant women, or patients with chronic illnesses.

Dry Brushing

Using natural dry brushes or shower gloves to exfoliate your skin right before the shower can be quite beneficial. This technique is derived from the age-old healing system of Ayurveda. It aids in the removal of dead skin cells, allowing the surface pores to open and act as a conduit for toxins to leave the body.

Massaging the skin also helps release toxins into the body's circulation, preparing them for elimination. After your shower, apply a great moisturizing organic body oil. This procedure is quick and simple and aids in internal and exterior detoxification. You take a step closer as soon as you buy brushes.

Souping

Souping involves consuming nutrient-dense, low-calorie hot or cold plant-based soups, and nourishing bone broths. It is sometimes referred to as "the new juicing." The preventive minerals and fiber found in soup act as the cleaning brush that removes potential toxins from the colon and is easier to absorb when consumed. The number of days you should eat mostly soup for nourishment largely depends on your plans.

Key Potential Advantages:

- Contrary to previous juice cleanses, souping provides fiber and a satisfying chew without exposing you to the sugar and desires that come with drinking conventional fruit juice.

- Since the fluids and fiber are filling, you won't feel hungry.

- Many people find it nearly impossible to consume just veggies, which have powerful anti-inflammatory and antioxidant properties. You can easily obtain all these advantages by eating soup.

Getting Enough Sleep

Medical professionals urge us to sleep for 7-9 hours at night, but many of us find it difficult to do so for a variety of reasons. According to a study, the distance between brain cells may widen during sleep, allowing fluid to flow more freely through the brain and flush away waste that accumulates during the day. These include harmful proteins linked to neurodegenerative illnesses like Alzheimer's, yet regular, quality sleep improves brain function.

Key Potential Advantages:

- Good sleep may help kill Alzheimer's.
- It helps to enhance mental alertness; reduces brain fog.

Spicing

Contrary to earlier times, Americans are now more accustomed to spices and purposefully utilize a wide range of these flavor enhancers when cooking. Additionally, there is a greater awareness of the health benefits of spices, which may help with detoxification. This is because many spices have anti-inflammatory and antioxidant properties that may allow detoxification organs like the liver and intestines to perform more effectively by reducing and eliminating inflammation.

You may provide your body with a steady supply of spices by getting five simple recipes that include them. There are several detoxifying spices available, some of which include black pepper, paprika, turmeric, and Ceylon cinnamon.

Key Potential Advantages:

- It doesn't need so many dietary changes, as long as you can spice up your existing meals.

- Spicing up the flavor of vegetables and other healthy grains can naturally enhance your consumption level on those meals.

Eliminating Problem Foods

Sometimes we encounter toxic overload symptoms; the elimination diet, also known as the "hypoallergenic diet," calls for giving up the most prevalent food in our diet for a month. You can get advice from a nutritionist on what to cut out; typically, cutting out gluten, soy, maize, dairy, sugar, and alcohol allows you to maintain a nutritious diet high in whole foods. The food you introduce after the order can then be used to determine the meal that appears unsuitable for your body system.

Key Potential Advantages:

- It gives a clue on what may be the cause of an adverse physical reaction in an individual.

- You can stop the excessive intake of sugar and processed foods that are causing diseases and any other adverse effect.

Cupping

Cupping was unknown prior to the 2016 Summer Olympics in Rio de Janeiro, but it came to public attention after some athletes—among them the renowned swimmer Michael Phelps—was seen sporting the technique's signature red circles on their skin. Because of this, cupping is now practiced and can be found on the menus of many spas and wellness centers.

This technique is related to traditional Chinese medicine, which uses small cups or jars on the skin to suction muscles and skin upward. With the help of this therapy, extra fluids and toxins are eliminated, adhesions and connective tissues are loose, and blood can circulate to tense muscles and skin. Cupping therapy is frequently combined with other traditional Chinese therapeutic techniques.

Key Potential Advantages:

- It frees up muscles and relaxes muscular pain and stiffness.

- It improves the digestion process.

- It calms the nervous system.

- It enhances the flow of blood and metabolic processes.

Practicing Yoga

The parasympathetic nervous system in your body can be brought under control by practicing deep rhythmic breathing as a yoga method. This promotes blood circulation and helps the body's metabolic process break down pollutants. The twisting positions, particularly the triangular pose, are all important parts of the detoxification process. Twisting postures remove obstructions in the lymph (the clear fluid of the lymphatic system that transports internal sludge to the lymph nodes for filtering) to enable the continuous flow. It is most often compared to wringing out a dirty sponge.

Key Potential Advantages:

- It helps keep your mind and body in a good state.

- Sweating can cause further detox.

- It can be done almost anywhere such as your home, studio, gym, field, etc.

Sweating

Although there is much uncertainty over the number of toxins expelled through sweat, much research supports regular, intense exercise and brief sessions in a steam room or sauna for detoxification. Researchers from Canada have discovered that sweating assists in the body's removal of several harmful substances.

Key Potential Advantages:

- You can choose your schedule, location before carrying out this activity.

- There are so much health-enhancing benefits of cardio at your fingertips.

Going Organic

Your exposure to pesticides, antibiotic-resistant germs, and hormones is decreased by choosing exclusively organic fruits, meats, vegetables, and dairy products, along with packaged goods bearing the USDA organic stamp. This decreases the stress on your body's natural detoxification mechanism. You can reduce your exposure to dangerous chemicals by eating only greens and using only items made from naturally cultivated ingredients.

Key Potential Advantages:

- A reduced contact with synthetic pesticides can further limit the rate of getting cancer, and for pregnant women, it reduces problems associated with brain development in their babies.

- It is a valid way to regulate the chemical intake we face on a daily basis.

Tongue Scraping

In your mouth, poisons develop throughout the night. Because of this, your tongue has a white coating when you wake up in the morning. This indicates that you have toxins in your body. You can remove harmful sludge every morning by scraping the tongue with a metal tongue cleaner by adhering to a straightforward daily Ayurvedic practice. About four times, drag the tongue cleaner down the tongue. You are removing toxins from the beginning of the digestive tract by doing this.

Key Potential Advantages:

- It gives you fresher breath by eliminating bacteria.

- It improves the taste receptors on the tongue.

- It immediately removes toxins.

BOOK 8
DR. SEBI APPROVED
HERBS PART II

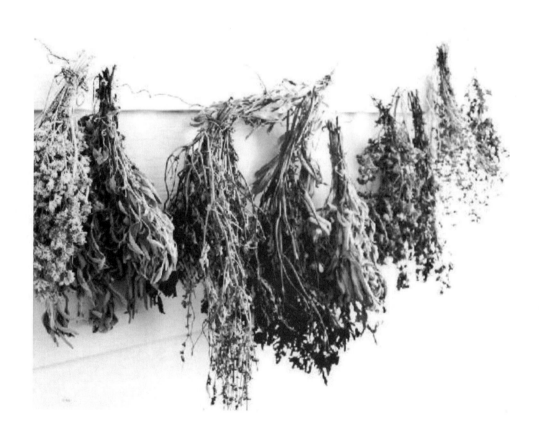

20 Herbs and Recipes

Basil

Overview

A herb with significant medical benefits is basil. For treating starch-related illnesses such as diarrhea, loss of appetite, intestinal gas, constipation, spasms, and other conditions, basil's upper section that grows above the ground is typically employed. It is claimed to have compounds that could kill germs and fungi; however, these claims are not yet supported by strong scientific evidence.

Benefits and Uses

Despite the need for additional scientific proof to support its claims, the following health issues it can help with are listed;

It aids in acne eradication.

It promotes mental clarity.

Head colds are decreased.

It makes you more hungry.

It aids in overcoming the problem of gas (flatulence).

It lessens stomach cramps.

It assists in treating diarrhea.

Constipation is fought off by it.

It makes your kidney stronger.

It guards against parasite infections in your intestine.

Warts are avoided.

Insect bites, etc., can be healed using it.

Contraindication

Eating basil with your mouth open is harmful because Estragole, which is present, can induce liver cancer. Basil should only be used in limited amounts in food since it contains the chemical Estragole, which negatively affects the liver.

An abnormal bleed can be caused by basil. Basil extracts and oils can decrease blood coagulation, which causes patients to bleed more frequently and develop bleeding disorders.

Blood pressure in the body can be lowered by using basil extracts.

NOTE: Due to the contraindications mentioned above, it is advisable for everyone, including children and pregnant women, to take basil in food in small quantities. Also, for surgical patients, it should be avoided due to it causing a bleeding disorder.

Recipe

Dr. Sebi's Basil Pesto "Zoodles'

This is a healthy meal containing basil pesto, cherry tomatoes, and combined with zucchini noodles. It can serve for both a dinner and a lunch dish.

Ingredients

Zucchini (small strips), 1 lb.

Grapeseed Oil, 1 tablespoon

Ripe Avocado, 1 Fruit

Packed Basil Leaves, ½ Cup

Walnuts, ¼ Cup

Olive Oil, ¼ Cup

Cayenne Pepper, ¼ Teaspoon

Cherry Tomatoes, 1 Cup

Juice from Lime, 1 Fruit

Sea Salt, ½ Teaspoon

Preparation

Sautee the zucchini noodles until it becomes soft but crunchy using grapeseed oil.

Put the rest ingredients inside a blender and blend them into a thick creamy paste.

Mix the paste and the already drained noodles, but if the dough is too thick, you can add water.

You can serve and garnish it with coconut.

Cayenne Pepper

Overview

Cayenne pepper is a member of the capsicum family. It is a spicy chile that people use to enhance the flavor of their food, and the nutrients it contains are also beneficial to their health. The bell pepper and jalapeno, which are stapled ingredients in Southern American, Mexican, Creole, Cajun, Korean, Sichuan, and other cuisines, are comparable to the cayenne pepper. It is pounded into a powder spice and sun-dried before being used as a condiment.

The cayenne pepper's spiciness is due to capsaicin, which is present in it. This is frequently used to treat aches and pains in muscles and joints. For this reason, cayenne pepper is used in traditional Chinese and Ayurvedic medicine to treat circulatory problems.

Uses and Benefits

Cayenne pepper has many advantages due to the presence of capsaicin, including the ability to ease the pain.

It supports the control of weight.

It lessens scratching.

It aids in lowering inflammation.

It assists in warding off congestion and colds.

It benefits and safeguards the nervous system.

Contraindication

Irritation of the digestive system may occur due to capsaicin.

People with both irritable bowel syndrome (IBS) and gastroesophageal reflux disease (GERD) should avoid cayenne pepper due to its spiciness.

Recipe

Dr. Sebi's Juicy Portobello Burgers

This meal can be a matchup with grains from Quinoa, Spelt or Kamut.

Ingredients

Large Portobello Mushroom, 2 Cups

Dried Basil, 2 Teaspoons

Dried Oregano, 1 Teaspoon

Olive Oil, 3 Tablespoons

Cayenne Pepper, ½ Teaspoon

Purslane, 1 Cup

Tomato, 1 Sliced

Avocado, 1 Sliced

Preparation

Chop off the stems of the mushrooms and cut ½ the top off the mushroom.

Put all the ingredients in a bowl, including the cayenne pepper and mix thoroughly.

Oil a foil and place on a cookie sheet, then place the mushroom cap on it.

Use a large spoon to pour marinade on each cap and leave it for about 10 minutes.

Ensure the oven is already pre-heated to 425°F, then bake the mushroom for about 10 minutes. Check it regularly to flip it for another 10 minutes.

Serve by placing the bottom of the mushroom on a plate and add your desired toppings, then cover with the upper part.

HEMP SEEDS

Overview

Although it is a member of the same species as cannabis, hemp contains less tetrahydrocannabinol. This quality makes it safe for use as a nutritional supplement and in food. Cannabis, cannabidiol, hemp agrimony, and Canadian hemp are not the same thing as hemp.

Uses

Here are some of the many applications for hemp seed;

It is utilized to create cosmetics.

It is utilized to create a textile.

Ropes are made from it.

It serves as a wood preserver.

As a lighting oil, it is utilized.

Detergents and soaps are made with it.

Ink for printers is made with it.

Health Benefits

With constipation, it aids.

It helps to reduce high cholesterol.

It aids in the skin's eczema removal.

It mitigates arthritis.

Blood pressure is lowered as a result.

It lessens swelling.

It facilitates bowel movements.

For people with asthma, it is beneficial.

Glaucoma is lessened by it.

Headaches are lessened.

This prevents cancer.

Menstrual cramps are lessened as a result.

It offers malaria protection.

Contraindication

Some persons can have an allergic reaction to hemp seed.

Not advisable for persons with low blood pressure, as it can also reduce blood pressure.

Surgical patients should avoid it.

Recipe

Detox Berry Smoothie

This drink is delightful and refreshing. It helps the body to remove unwanted toxins from inside out.

Ingredients

Burro Banana, 1 Medium Size

Seville Orange, 1 Fruit

Berries (a mixture of blue, rasp, and strawberries or only blueberries), 1 Cup

Fresh Lettuce, 2 Cups

Water

¼ Avocado

Hemp Seeds, 1 Tablespoon

Preparation

Pour water into the blender and add the fruits and vegetables.

Blend all of them until it becomes smooth and enjoy your smoothie.

Fennel

Overview

Fennel is a lovely plant with yellow coloring, a pleasant aroma, and perpetual blossoms. It is currently grown all across the world. It is primarily found in the Mediterranean, though it shares some traits with anise. The seeds are used as a spice in cooking after being dried and combined with oil to take medication. While not all fennel's uses and health advantages are supported by scientific research, some are given here.

Uses

It is applied to a variety of stomach problems.

To stop women's excessive hair growth, it is applied topically.

Additionally, flavoring agents employ it.

In cosmetics and soap, it serves as a scent.

Health Benefits

It eases menstruation discomfort.

It aids in easing menopausal symptoms.

This lessens sunburn.

It eases vaginal thinning symptoms such as discomfort, dryness, and itching during sexual activity.

Irritable bowel syndrome is alleviated (IBS).

Intestinal gas, constipation, cough, bloating, moderate spasms, upset stomach, and upper respiratory infection are all helped by it.

Contraindications

Nursing moms should not consume fennel since it may harm the baby's neurological system.

For those sensitive to mugwort, carrot, and celery, it could exacerbate their allergy.

Fennel may make bleeding disorders worse.

By functioning like oestrogen, it can make some illnesses worse.

Recipe

Dr. Sebi's Herbal Smoothie

It was over 4000 years ago that herbs were first documented to remove pathologies. This meal brings ancient healing tea to the modern age.

Ingredients

Fennel Herbs

Walnuts, 1 Tablespoon

Burro Banana, 1 Lump

Agave Syrup or Date Sugar, 1 Tablespoon

Preparation

Prepare the fennel tea as instructed in the package instructions and allow to cool.

Pour water into the blender and add all the ingredients, then blend properly until it forms a perfect mix.

Pour in a cup and enjoy.

Quinoa

Overview

Quinoa is a seed-bearing plant, and the seeds are consumed similarly to grains like wheat. Although it has similar characteristics to grains, it differs because it has more protein than conventional grains. Additionally, gluten is not present in it.

Compared to those who eat normal grains like rice, those who eat quinoa report feeling fuller. Quinoa offers a lower blood fat supply than bread (triglycerides).

Uses

It is employed to make flour.

For those with celiac disease or other dietary restrictions to gluten, it can be used in place of wheat.

Soups are made using it.

To make beer, it is used.

Health Benefits

Some of the health advantages that have been the subject of speculation include the reduction of blood sugar, blood pressure, and blood fat in obese men and postmenopausal women.

In the fight against celiac disease.

It has the ability to repel insects.

It lessens discomfort.

Urinary tract infections are helped by it.

Contraindication

Amaranth can trigger an allergy in people allergic to grains.

Pregnant and breastfeeding mothers should avoid amaranth because the side effects are not fully known yet.

Recipe

Dr. Sebi's Blueberry Smoothie

This meal is highly nutritious and delicious. You can have it for breakfast, and you are sure of being refreshed and energized.

Ingredients

Cooked Quinoa, 1 Cup

Blueberries, ½ Cup

Homemade Walnut Milk, 1 Cup

Burro Banana, 1 Lump

Date Sugar, 2 Tablespoons

Preparation

Pour water into a blender and add all the ingredients.

Blend them on high speed until it becomes a paste.

Serve and enjoy your smoothie.

Plant-Based Quinoa Bowl

This is an easy meal to cook, and it is also a delicious and filling dish. A perfect recipe for your lunch and dinner.

Ingredients

Cooked Quinoa, 1 Cup

Dandelion Greens, 1 Handful

Grapeseed Oil, 1 Tablespoon

Chopped Cherry Tomatoes, 2 Cups

Cayenne Pepper to taste

Sea Salt to taste

Preparation

Pour all the grapeseed oil into a large pan and sauté the chopped cherry tomatoes until it becomes soft.

Combine the dandelion greens, cherry tomatoes, and cooked quinoa and mix thoroughly.

Add both the cayenne pepper and sea salt to season it to taste.

Amaranth

Overview

The seeds, leaves, and oil of the amaranth plant are all edible as well as being very therapeutic. It is useful and has several health advantages. Some of the compounds it contains exhibit antioxidant-like behaviours.

Uses

Amaranth is used as a pseudo cereal.

Benefits

Amaranth aids in regulating the body's cholesterol levels.

It guards against gastric ulcers.

It also aids in the prevention of diarrhea.

It reduces tongue and throat swelling.

Contraindication

Since the sides effect are not established yet, it is safer for pregnant breastfeeding women to avoid amaranth.

Recipe

Dr. Sebi's Sleepy Time drink

Most persons find it difficult to sleep, maybe due to one issues or the other. But this recipe will help knock you ought, and it is tasty to sip and relax.

Ingredients

Cooked Quinoa, ¼ Cup

Amaranth Greens, 2 Cups

Dr. Sebi's Nerve Relief Herbal Tea, ½ Cup

Dr. Sebi's Stomach Relief Herbal Tea, ½ Cup

Burro Banana, 1 Lump

Cherries, ¼ Cup

Agave syrup to taste

Preparation

Prepare both the stomach relief and nerve relief tea according to the packaged specifications and allow it to cool.

Pour water into a blender and add all the ingredients, blend them properly until it becomes smooth.

Pour into a cup and enjoy your drink.

Habanero (chili pepper)

Overview

The habanero is a member of the Chinese capsicum family and is often known as red pepper or chili pepper. In addition to being used to make medicine, it also has several health benefits, some of which are listed below:

Uses

It can be used as pepper spray for self-defense.

Health Benefits

People with diabetes who experience nerve pain benefit from its painkilling properties.

It helps relieve psoriasis, rheumatoid arthritis, jaw discomfort, and other types of pain.

It lessens and restores nerve damage brought on by shingles.

When applied with a plaster, back discomfort is significantly reduced.

It lessens the effects of osteoarthritis.

The direct application is also used to stop running noses.

When used before surgery, it lowers the need for painkillers.

When utilized, it improves athletes' performance.

Blood sugar levels are lowered by it, particularly in pregnant women who have gestational diabetes.

It lessens heartburn and indigestion.

It benefits obese people and lowers the risk of ulcers.

Contraindications

It should not be taken in excess since it may irritate and upset the stomach.

When applying it to the skin, the eyes should be covered to prevent eye irritation.

Because it can cause dermatitis, nursing mothers should take precautions to prevent their infants from coming into contact with it.

Applying to skin that has been injured is not advised.

Recipe

Plant-Based Fajitas Taco

This meal is a Mexican dinner, rich in flavor and fast to prepare. If you love tacos, you can go on to try these plant-based fajitas tacos.

Ingredients

Portobello Mushrooms, 2-3 large sized ones

Bell peppers, 2 Fruits

Onion, 1 Bulb

Lime Juice, ½ Size

Grapeseed Oil, 1 Tablespoon

Kamut Flour Tortillas, 6

Habanero

Avocado

Preparation

Wash the mushroom properly and slice into reasonable sizes.

Slice both the onions and bell peppers.

Pour the grapeseed oil into a skillet and cook the pepper and onions for about 2 minutes.

Pour in the seasonings and mushroom and stir regularly, allow to cook for about 7-8 minutes.

Heat the tortillas to warm and spread the fajitas mix in the center.

Serve along with key lime juice and avocado.

Onion

Overview

The onion is a vital plant for cooking, and it is used everywhere in the world. It also has medicinal benefits.

Uses

It is used for scarring.

It is used for other skin conditions, and also to prevent cancer and heart disease.

Health Benefits

It has compounds that aid in reducing inflammation.

It aids people with asthma in lessening tightness in their lungs.

Reduced hair loss is a result.

Patients who have diabetes can benefit from it.

It lessens the chance of stomach and prostate cancer.

Contraindication

It might lead to stomach distress if taken in too much quantity.

There is a tendency it might slow blood clots.

Recipe

Mushroom Risotto

This meal is very creamy, rich, and full of flavor. It is a perfect meal for dinner.

Ingredients

Grapeseed Oil, 1 Tablespoon

Mushrooms, 4 Lumps

Onion, ½ Bulb

Wild Rice, 2 Cups

Homemade Vegetable Broth, 4 Cups

Cayenne Pepper to taste

Sea Salt to taste

Preparation

Pour the grapeseed oil in a big pot, sauté the onion and mushrooms on medium heat. Cook until the mushrooms become brown or for about 7 minutes, while stirring it regularly.

Pour in the rice and continue cooking for another minute.

Add the cayenne pepper, sea salt and vegetable broth. Cover the pot and allow it to cook for about 3 hours on low heat or 1 hour 30 minutes on high heat, or until the rice becomes soft.

Oregano

Overview

An herb from the Lamiaceae family is oregano (mint). Oregano has a long history; the Romans and the Greeks associated it with joy and happiness thousands of years ago. It has several uses and advantageous effects on health.

Uses

In tropical locations, it is employed to deter insects.

In foods and beverages, it serves as a spice and preservative.

Health Benefits

Asthma, bronchitis, and other respiratory tract diseases are all improved by it.

It assists ladies with menstruation cramps and rheumatoid arthritis.

Additionally, it lessens urethral tract infections.

It eases headache pain.

It helps with the relief of digestive issues like bloating and heartburn.

It aids in the removal of athlete's foot, ringworm, warts, acne, and other skin conditions when administered to the skin.

Insect bites, muscle aches, toothaches, gum disease, and other conditions are also helped by it.

It has compounds that lessen coughing and spasms.

Assists with digestion.

Contraindication

If eaten in excess, it might upset your stomach.

Those allergic to members of the Lamiaceae family may experience allergic responses.

Recipe

Magic Green Falafel

This is a delicious alkaline-flavored dish, and it is fast and easy.

Ingredients

Dry Garbanzo Beans (Chickpeas), 2 Cups

Chopped Onion, 1 Large Bulb

Chopped Red Bell Pepper, 1/3 Cup

Fresh Dill, ½ Cup

Fresh Basil, 2/3 Cup

Garbanzo Bean Flour, ½ Cup

Oregano, ¼ Teaspoon

Avocado or Grapeseed Oil for frying

Sea Salt, 1 Teaspoon

Preparation

Cook the chickpeas until it becomes tender, and then drain and rinse the beans.

Place all the ingredients in a food processor and add the chickpeas.

Power the processor and slice the ingredients until they become finely chopped.

Pour the mix into a bowl. Form small balls with your hands and place them in a paper parchment.

Place inside the refrigerator and cool for about an hour.

Pour oil into a big skillet to a reasonable depth, and heat on medium heat for about 7 minutes—Fry the magic green falafel in the hot oil 3 minutes on each side.

Wild Arugula

Overview

The kale, cabbage, and broccoli families are all closely related to arugula (Eruca Vesicaria). It is a cruciferous vegetable with spicy, peppery leaves that become increasingly bitter over time. It has edible seeds and can be used to create oil. A milder kind called baby arugula is sold in supermarkets, but regular arugula has a strong flavor. Early harvesting by farmers results in very nutritious crops that are also mineral-rich. Fat, sodium, carbs, protein, vitamins, magnesium, and potassium are a few of these.

Uses

There are a variety of applications for arugula, some of which are listed below;

Pasta is made using it.

In salads, it is utilized.

In sandwiches, it is used in place of lettuce.

It is put in omelets or smoothies.

It's utilized in soups and sauces.

It is used as a topping on pizza or baked potatoes.

Health Benefits

It can either prevent or repair cell damage.

It guards against prostate, colon, lung, and breast cancer.

It reduces inflammation.

It guards against osteoporosis.

Contraindication

When taking blood thinners, stay away from arugula because too much vitamin K can impair it.

Recipe

Detox Salad Burritos

Detox salad burritos is a quick fix meal wrapped up in tortillas. A healthy veggie dish to satisfy you.

Ingredients

Wild Arugula, 2 Cups

Cherry Tomatoes, 2 Cups

Homemade Fresh Sesame "tahini" butter, 2 Tablespoons

Garbanzo Beans (Cooked Chickpeas), 1 Cup

Kamut Flour Tortillas, 4

Key Lime Juice, 1 Tablespoon

Cayenne Pepper to taste

Sea Salt to taste

Preparation

Place the key lime juice and tahini butter in a small cup and whisk.

Pour the cherry tomatoes, chickpeas, and wild arugula in a big bowl and mix thoroughly. Add the dressing on top to cover it and place in the refrigerator for 20 minutes.

Place the kamut flour tortillas on a big pan and warm up over low heat.

Put the salad inside the tortillas to fill it, add your cayenne pepper and sea salt, and then roll up and enjoy your meal.

Red Onion

Overview

There are varieties of onion called red onions, which have purplish-red skin and white flesh. This onion has an eye-watering trait and a pungent flavour, just like other species.

Uses

You can use red onions as a dye.

It can also be employed in cooking.

Health Benefits

It has compounds that aid in reducing inflammation.

It aids people with asthma in lessening tightness in their lungs.

Reduced hair loss is a result.

Patients who have diabetes can benefit from it.

It lessens the chance of stomach and prostate cancer.

Contraindication

If consumed in excess, it could cause gastrointestinal discomfort.

There is a chance that it could prevent blood clots.

Recipe

Dr. Sebi's Mango Salad

This is a versatile, slightly spicy and sweet, full of flavor, and fresh meal.

Ingredients

Mangoes, 2 Fruit

Red Onion, ¼ bulbs

Seeded Cucumber, ½

Cherry Tomatoes, ½ Cup

Green Bell Pepper, ½

Key Lime, ½

Cayenne Pepper to taste

Sea Salt to taste

Preparation

Dice the cherry tomatoes, red onion bulbs, and mangoes into tiny cubes.

Finely slice the green bell pepper and seeded cucumber.

Pour all the ingredients into a bowl and mix them thoroughly. Juice the key lime and add it to the mix.

Add the cayenne pepper and sea salt and put in the refrigerator for 20 minutes.

Enjoy your salad.

Tea Plant

Overview

Green tea, oolong tea, and black tea are all produced by the tea plant (Camellia sinensis). Although the leaves from the tea plant are used to make these teas, the method is what distinguishes them. Black and oolong teas go through fermentation and partial fermentation. In contrast, green tea is made by pan-frying and boiling the tea leaves.

Uses

Genital warts may be treated with a prescription for it.

It is a vitamin that can help burn extra fat and lower cholesterol levels.

Health Benefits

It lessens the risk of cardiac problems.

Endometrial cancer risk is decreased.

Parkinson's disease risk is also decreased.

Contraindication

It can lead to constipation or stomach upset when taken continuously for a long time.

It also triggers headache, irritability, dizziness, heartburn, sleeping problems, and vomiting, etc.

Recipe

Mood-Boosting Smoothie

This smoothie amazingly possesses the ability to lighten your mood and make you feel good.

Ingredients

Tea Plant (Green Tea), 1 Cup

Soft-Jelly Coconut Meat, ½ Cup

Strawberries, 1 Cup

Agave Syrup or Date Sugar, to taste

Preparation

Prepare the tea as specified in the packaged instruction.

Pour the tea and all the ingredients into a blender and blend on high speed.

Serve and enjoy your smoothie.

Dill

Overview

Dill is the only plant species in the genus Anethum, a member of the celery family (Apiaceae). Dill is a perennial plant that grows widely in Asia and Europe. The leaves are used as herbs and spices.

Uses

It is employed as a cooking spice.

It serves as a scent for soaps and cosmetics.

It also has therapeutic uses.

Health Benefits

It lessens the discomfort of period cramps.

On the skin, it has an anti-aging effect.

Among other things, it aids in the fight against cough, fever, colds, bronchitis, digestive system issues, infections, liver issues, and spasms.

Contraindication

It has anti-allergic qualities.

It could cause skin irritation.

Dill should be avoided by expectant mothers because it can cause miscarriage.

Recipe

Cherry Tomato Salad

This is the perfect side dish for your family. It is filled with flavor, and is fresh, and healthy.

Ingredients

Cherry Tomatoes, 4 Cups

Chopped Red Onion, ¼ Cup

Fresh Dill, ¼ Cup

Key Lime Juice. 1½ Tablespoons

Olive Oil, ¼ Cup

Date Sugar, ¼ Teaspoon

Cayenne Pepper, to taste

Sea Salt, to taste

Preparation

Pour the herbs, red onion, and cherry tomatoes in a big bowl.

Mix the key lime juice, olive oil, date sugar, cayenne pepper, and sea salt in a smaller bowl.

Place the dressing on the tomato mixture and carefully spread to coat evenly.

Serve and enjoy your salad.

Cloves

Overview

Syzygium aromaticum, or cloves, are a member of the Myrtaceae family. Although it originated in Indonesia's Maluku Islands, it is currently grown in South America.

Uses

It is used to flavor dishes and drinks.

It is a component in producing toothpaste, cigarettes, cosmetics, and perfumes.

It functions as a mosquito repellent.

Health Benefits

Anal fissure healing is aided by it.

It lessens discomfort.

It relieves itching.

It eases dental discomfort.

Bad breath is avoided.

Additionally, it relieves gas and indigestion.

Contraindication

Lung disease and respiratory problems may result from it.

It may result in burning and skin irritation.

Recipe

Alkaline-Electric Classic Apple Bake

This is a combo of sweet, tart, and fresh apple and some healthy spices.

Ingredient

Honeycrisp or Gala Apples, 3-4 Fruits

Agave Syrup, 3 Tablespoons

Chopped Walnuts, 1 Tablespoon

Cloves, a pinch

Preparation

Preheat the oven to about 350 degrees. Then, slice the apples into small sizes and pour them into a big bowl. Drizzle it with agave syrup and stir it very well to coat properly.

Mix the cloves and walnuts, and then spread over the agave coated apples. Continue to stir and allow it to settle for 5 minutes.

Place the sliced apples orderly in a casserole dish.

Bake for about 15 minutes, remove and wrap in a foil, then bake again for about 40 minutes or until the aroma fills the kitchen and the apples become bubbly.

Dried Thyme

Overview

One of the most popular herbs in the world is thyme. Thyme's oil, leaves, and flowers are its main therapeutic components, while it can also be used in combination with other herbs.

Uses

It serves as an anti-irritant for the skin.

Bad breath is treated with it.

It is applied to stop tooth decay.

It's employed to treat baldness.

It is employed in mouthwash as an antiseptic.

Foods are flavored with it.

It is a component in producing toothpaste, soap, fragrances, and other goods.

Health Benefits

Thyme oil is effective in combating dyspraxia.

It aids in easing bronchitis symptoms.

It lessens coughing, especially in bronchitis sufferers.

The sore throat is avoided.

It stops the tonsils from the swell.

Contraindication

When ingested in excess, it may cause headaches, nausea, or digestive problems.

For those who are allergic to oregano, it may cause an allergic reaction.

Estrogen may be triggered by it.

Recipes

Dr. Sebi's Chickpea Loaf

This meal is not your regular meatloaf, but it is sweeter. Chickpea loaf is baked to perfection with a seasoned chickpeas base.

Ingredients

Finely Diced Onions, 1½ Cups

Bell Pepper, 2 finely diced

Minced Fresh Basil, ½ Cup

Grapeseed Oil, 2 Tablespoons

Homemade Natural Granulated Onion, 2 Tablespoons and ½ Teaspoon

Dried Sage, ¾ Teaspoon

Dried Oregano, ½ Teaspoon

Sea Salt, 1 Teaspoon

Cayenne Pepper, ½ Teaspoon

Dried Thyme, ¼ Teaspoon

Cooked Chickpeas, 3 Cups

Mushroom, 1 Cup

Spelt Flour, ½ Cup

Cayenne Pepper, to taste

Sea Salt, to taste

Preparation

Ensure the oven is preheated to 350°F.

Pour the grapeseed oil into a big pan and heat on medium heat. Then add the bell pepper and mushroom, and sauté.

Mix it with the minced basil and carry it off the heat. Mix the seasonings and pour them into the mixture.

Either slice the chickpeas or use a food processor to chop it. Mix and pour into the sautéed vegetables, and you can add spelt flour and mix thoroughly.

Rub grease on the loaf pan and bake at 350°F for about an hour without covering it.

Bell Pepper

Overview

The bell peppers, commonly known as capsicum annuum, are members of the nightshade family. The bell pepper has ties to chili peppers, tomatoes, and breadfruit. It is a plant that grows in central and south America and is frequently called sweet pepper. You can eat it cooked or uncooked, dry it out and grind it into paprika.

Uses

It speeds up hair growth.

You can use it to make your skin glow.

Health Benefits

It lowers the chance of developing cancer.

It shields the eye against illnesses.

It guards against anaemia.

Contraindication

It tends to be allergenic.

It could result in cross-reactivity.

Recipe

Tef Grain Burgers

Ingredients

Cooked Tef Grains, 1½ Cups

Garbanzo Beans, 1½ Cups

Diced Onion, ¼ Bulb

Finely Diced Bell Peppers, ¼ Cup

Basil, 1 Teaspoon

Oregano, 1Teaspoon

Dill, 1 Teaspoon

Grapeseed Oil, 1 Tablespoon

Cayenne Pepper, to taste

Sea Salt, to taste

Preparation

Turn the grapeseed oil into a frying pan and add your pepper and onions, then sauté until it becomes soft.

Pour the ingredients and the vegetables (sautéed) into a big bowl and mix.

Use your hands to form patties and place them in the skillet to cook for 3 minutes on both sides.

When it becomes crisp, serve and enjoy.

Dandelion Greens

Overview

This herb is mainly found in mild climatic conditions and is native to Europe.

Dandelion green is a herb used for numerous purposes, as highlighted below.

Uses

They can be used to make wine.

They can be utilised as food flavouring.

Health Benefits

It aids in lowering inflammation.

It aids in the prevention of urinary tract infections.

It stimulates hunger.

This avoids constipation.

Contraindication

An allergic response could result.

It might cause abdominal discomfort.

It might lead to heartburn.

Diarrhea may also result from it.

Recipe

Heart-Healthy Smoothie

Ingredients

Organic or Braeburn Apple, 1 Fruit

Brazil Nuts, ¼ Cup

Homemade Walnut Milk, 1 Cup

Dandelion Greens, 1 Cup

Blueberries, 1 Cup

Agave Syrup, ½ Tablespoon

Preparation

Pour all the ingredients into a blender, and blend them to paste.

Serve and enjoy your smoothie.

Watercress

Overview

Watercress, commonly known as yellowcress, is a member of the cabbage family (Brassicaceae). It is one of the earliest vegetable leaves consumed by humans and is a perennial in Asia and Europe.

Uses

As a salad, it is used.

It is also employed as a spice in cooking.

Health Benefits

It eliminates recent inflammation.

It stops balding.

Contraindication

It could cause an uncomfortable stomach.

Patients with ulcers should avoid watercress.

People with kidney problems should also stay away from it.

Recipe

Detox Watercress Citrus Salad

This diet is a very rich and refreshing dish, and it has numerous antioxidants and nutrients to protect and build the body.

Ingredients

Ripe Avocado, 1 Fruit

Watercress, 4 Cups

Zested, Peeled, and Sliced Seville Orange, 1 Fruit

Red Onion, 2 Thin Slices

Agave Syrup, 2 Teaspoons

Key Lime Juice, 2 Tablespoons

Olive Oil, 2 Tablespoons

Salt, 1/8 Teaspoon

Cayenne Pepper.

Preparation

Correctly place the oranges, watercress, avocado and onion on two separate plates.

Pour the olive, oil, agave syrup, key lime juice, cayenne pepper, and salt into a bowl and mix thoroughly.

Use a spoon to spread the mix on the salad and enjoy your meal.

Cherry Tomato

Overview

One of the plants that is most commonly consumed worldwide is this one. It has therapeutic advantages in addition to flavour and pleasant taste in food.

Uses

It can be used as a meal garnish.

You can use it to make sauce.

Health Benefits

Reduces high blood pressure

Additionally, it aids in the battle against cancer.

It helps people with diabetes.

Contraindication

If not used with prudence, it may cause food poisoning.

It could cause throat and mouth irritation.

It might result in death.

Recipe

Zoodles with Avocado Sauce

Ingredients

Zucchini, 2 Large

Basil, 2 Cups

Water, ½ Cup

Walnuts, ½ Cup

Cherry Tomatoes, 24 Sliced

Avocados, 2 Fruits

Key Lime Juice, 4 Tablespoons

Sea Salt, to taste

Preparation

Use a spiralizer or peeler to prepare the zucchini.

Properly blend all the ingredients in a blender, except the cherry tomato.

Mix the sliced cherry tomatoes, avocado sauce, and the noodles in a bowl.

Serve and enjoy the meal.

Raspberry

Overview

Raspberry is a fruity plant that has multi-purpose functions. For centuries, it has been a good source of medicine.

Uses

It helps pregnant women during labor.

It is applied to treat skin rashes.

Jams can be made using it.

Additionally, it is utilized to flavor meals.

Health Benefits

Patients with diabetes can benefit from it.

It combats gastrointestinal illnesses.

It guards against cardiac disorders.

It gives the body vitamins.

Contraindication

Due to the presence of estrogen, a doctor should closely supervise raspberry consumption for pregnant women.

Recipe

Dr. Sebi's Triple Berry Smoothie

Ingredients

Strawberries, ½ Cup

Raspberry, ½ Cup

Blueberry, ½ Cup

Water, 1 Cup

Burro Banana, 1 Lump

Agave Syrup, to taste

Preparation

Pour all the ingredients into a blender, and blend them until they form a paste.

Pour in a cup and enjoy.

BOOK 8
Dr. Sebi's Recipes

200 Delicious and Simple Recipes to Naturally Cleanse Your Liver, Lose Weight, and Lower High Blood Pressure, And Improve your health by detoxifying your body with an alkaline diet.

Salads:
20 Recipes

Onion Avocado Salad

Ingredients

- 1 avocado diced or cut into small pieces 6 to 8 plum or cherry tomatoes, sliced or diced

- 2 medium-sized onions, Iced or diced

- 1/2 teaspoon cayenne pepper

- A pinch of sea salt (optional)

- 1/2 teaspoon cayenne pepper

- 1 teaspoon lime juice (optional)

Instructions:

In a bowl, combine the onion, avocado, and tomato and mix well.

Add lime juice, cayenne, and sea salt and toss.

The salad can be eaten alone or with vegetables, cooked unoa, puffed dumplings, or other alternatives of your choice.

Onion Avocado Dip

Onion Avocado Dip: Ingredients

- 3 medium-sized onions, chopped
- 1 teaspoon olive oil (optional)
- 1 avocado, chopped
- 8 plum or cherry tomatoes
- 1/2 teaspoon cayenne pepper
- Juice of 1 medium-sized orange
- 1 tablespoon fresh herbs
- 1/2 teaspoon salt

Onion Avocado Dip: Instructions:

- Place all ingredients in a blender or food processor and mix until smooth.
- Chill and serve.

Onion Avocado Dip: Pairing suggestions

- General dip
- Instead of gravy, use over food.
- Pour over salad
- Blend with le orange juice to make it firmer and use instead of spread.

Note: Do not keep for more than 1 day as it may go bad quickly because avocado and tomatoes do not last long once used.

Roasted Quinoa Salad

Ingredients:

- 2 green bell peppers, sliced lengthwise
- 2 ½ cups vegetable homemade broth
- 2 cups quinoa
- 2 teaspoons sea salt
- 2 tablespoons grapeseed oil
- Red bell pepper, cored and diced
- Cut up zucchini into bite-sized pieces
- 3 cups wild arugula
- Sea salt
- Red onion, to taste.
- 1 avocado

Instructions:

- Preheat oven to 400 degrees.
- Bring the broth and salt to a boil over medium heat, then stir in the unoa. Stir well to bring the quinoa to a low simmer, then reduce the heat to low and cover. Allow it simmer for 20 minutes, then turn off the heat and set aside until ready to serve. Just before serving, fluff the unoa with a fork.
- Toss together then garnish with onion and avocado as you fold in the q uinoa.
- While the unoa is simmering, add the bell peppers and zucchini to a sheet pan and toss with olive oil and sea salt to taste. Bake for 10-12 minutes, or until everything is golden and tender.

Summer Quinoa Salad

Ingredients:

- 1 red bell pepper, finely diced
- 3 ½ cups veggie broth
- 2 cup raw quinoa, cleaned
- ½ cup red onion, finely chopped
- 3/4 cup roughly chopped dried cranberries
- 1 cup cilantro, chopped
- 1-2 avocados, diced

Dressing:

- ¼ tsp. cayenne pepper (optional)
- 1/3 cup red wine vinegar
- 2 T. olive oil
- 2 T. Dijon mustard
- ½ tsp. sea salt
- 1 T. raw agave nectar

Instructions:

- Add uinoa, vegetable broth, and a pinch of salt to a small pot, cover, and bring to a boil.
- Reduce heat to medium-low, open the lid slightly to let some steam to escape, and simmer until all of the liquid has been absorbed.
- Remove from heat, fluff with a fork, and place in a bowl to cool.
- Whisk the dressing ingredients together.
- When the quinoa has completely cooled, whisk in the remaining ngredent along with the dreng.
- Serve and enjoy.

Dr. Sebi's Asian Cucumber Salad

Do you think you know what cucumbers are all about? Try the Asian Cucumber Salad, and you'll be pleasantly surprised at how much better they can be.

Ingredients:

- 1 tbs. sesame oil
- 3 tbs. key lime juice
- 1 tbs. sesame seeds
- 1/2 tsp. date sugar
- 1 tbs. powdered granulated seaweed
- 1/4 tsp. sea salt
- 1 tbs. grated ginger

Instructions

To prepare your Aan Cucumber Salad, simply combine everything and serve!

Dr. Sebi's Mango Salad

Are you attempting to eat eaonally? Dr. Sebi's Mango Salad is veratle, freh, a bit spicy, a touch sweet, and bursting with flavour.

Ingredients:

- 2 mangoes
- 1/4 cup cherry tomatoes
- 1/4 red onion
- 1 key lime
- 1/2 cucumber, seeded
- To taste, sea salt and cayenne pepper.
- 1/2 green bell pepper

Instructions:

- Begin by chopping the mangoes, cherry tomatoes, and red on n tiny cube to make your Mango Salad.
- Slice the seeded cucumber and the bell pepper finely.
- Mix all of the ingredients in a large bowl. Spritz the key lime over the salad.
- Season with sea salt and pepper and set aside in the fridge for at least 20 minutes before serving.
- Enjoy as a salad, salsa, or dip, it's your call!

Cherry Tomato Salad

Prepare to serve the Cherry Tomato Salad to your family all summer long! The savoury side dh healthy, freh, alkalne-electrc, and flavorful!

Ingredients:

- 4 cups cherry tomatoes

- 1/4 cup fresh (approved) herbs, like dill, sweet basil, or thyme

- 1/4 cup red onion, chopped

- 1/2 tablespoons key lime juice

- 1/4 cup olive oil

- To taste, add salt and cayenne pepper.

- 1/4 teaspoon date sugar

Instructions:

- To prepare your cherry tomato alad, place the tomatoes, red onion, and herb n a large bowl.

- Now, let's get the party started! To taste, combine the olive oil, lime juice, date ugar, sea salt, and cayenne pepper in a small bowl.

- Pour the dressing over the tomato mixture and gently toss to coat evenly. Serve, and enjoy!

Detox Salad Burritos

A quick and easy salad wrapped in approved-grain tortillas for when your diet needs a reset. Green and vegetable in a healthy-burrtto form! A simple, fresh Detox Salad Burrtto.

Ingredients:

- 2 cups wild arugula, or other greens of choice

- 1 tablespoon key lime juice

- 2 cups cherry tomatoes

- Homemade raw eame "tahini" butter 2 tablepoon

- 4 Kamut flour tortillas

- 1 cup cooked chickpeas (garbanzo beans)

- To taste, sea salt and cayenne pepper

Instructions:

- Prepare the dressing in a small cup by whisking together key lime juice and raw sesame "tahn" butter. Set aside.

- In a large mixing basin, combine arugula, cherry tomatoes, and chickpeas. Cover with the dreng and let aside for 20 minutes in the refrigerator.

- Warm the Kamut flour tortillas on a large pan or griddle over low heat until they are ready.

- Fill the tortillas with the salad, season with sea salt and cayenne pepper, and roll-up. Enjoy!

Alkaline-Electric Spring Salad

Eating eaonal frut and vegetable is a fantastic way to care for yourself and the environment at the same time. The alkaline-electric alad is tasty, healthful, and environmentally friendly.

Ingredients:

- 4 cup sea seasonally approved green of your choice (wild arugula, dandelon green, watercress)

- 1/4 cup of your favourite herbs (dill, weet basil, etc.)

- 1/4 cup walnuts

- 1 cup cherry tomatoes

For The Dressing:

- 3-4 key limes

- Sea salt and cayenne pepper, to taste

- 1 tablespoon of homemade raw sesame "tahini" butter

Instructions:

Juice the key limes.

In a small bowl, combine the key lime juice and the homemade raw almond butter. To taste, add more salt and cayenne pepper.

Cut the cherry tomatoes in half.

Combine the green, cherry tomatoe, and herb in a large basin. Place the dress on top and "rub" it with your hand.

Let the greens soak up the dressing. Add more sea salt, cayenne pepper, and herbs on top if you wish. Enjoy!

Dr. Sebi's Chickpea Loaf

The hearty, alkaline-electric, plant-baed "meatloaf" created from a bae of eaoned chckpea baked to perfection. This Checkpea Loaf is superior than a traditional "meatloaf."

Ingredients:

- 2 bell peppers, finely diced
- 1/2 cups of finely diced onions
- 1/2 cup minced fresh basil
- 2 tablespoons grapeseed oil
- 1/2 teaspoon cayenne pepper
- 2 tablespoons + 1/2 teaspoon homemade natural granulated onion
- 1 teaspoon of sea salt
- 3/4 teaspoon dried sage
- 1/4 teaspoon dried thyme
- 1/2 teaspoon dried oregano
- 1 cup mushrooms (all kinds, except shiitake)
- 1/2 cup spelled flour
- 3 cups chickpeas, cooked
- Sea salt and cayenne pepper, to taste

Instructions:

Preheat oven to 350°F.

Sauté the mushroom, bell pepper, and onion in grapeed ol in a big pan over medium-high heat for 2 to 3 minutes.

Stir in minced basil and remove from heat. Stir in seasonings.

Carefully chop the chcckpea in a food processor or by hand. Str into cooked veggies. Mix with the pelleted flour.

Grease a loaf pan with grapeeed ol. Bake uncovered for 55 to 60 minutes at 350°F.

Nori-Burritos

These alkaline-electric eaweed rolls are packed with alkaline-electric, potent nourishment. We are confident that you will enjoy the new wrap!

Ingredients:

- 450 gr. cucumber (seeded)

- 1 avocado, ripe

- 4 sheets nori seaweed

- 1/2 mango, ripe

- 1 tbs. tahini

- 1 zucchini, small

- Handful amaranth or dandelon greens

- A handful of hemp seeds prouted

- Sesame seeds, to taste

Instructions:

- Place the Nori heet, hny side down, on a cutting board.

- Arrange all of the ngredents on the nor heet, leaving a nch ware margin of uncovered nor to the rght.

- Using both hands, fold the heet of nor from the edge closest to you, folding it up and over the filling.

- Cut in thick slices and sprinkle with sesame seeds.

- This Nori Roll would go well with a Wakame Salad.

Headache Preventing Salad

Due to their high odum content, most bottled drinks might cause headaches. The salad contains solely whole, natural ingredients. Prevent headaches with this healthful, refreshing salad.

Ingredients:

- 2 tbsp. olive oil

- 1/2 seeded cucumber

- 1 tbsp key lime juice

- 2 cups watercress
- To taste, season with salt and cayenne pepper.

Instructions:

Mix the olive oil and key lime until thoroughly blended.

Arrange watercre and cucumber

Add the dreng and sprinkle with salt and pepper to taste.

Detox Watercress Citrus Salad

The Watercree Citrus Salad is extremely nutritious, packed with antioxidants and minerals, and both refreshing and tasty.

Ingredients:

- 4 cups watercress
- 1 avocado, ripe
- 1 Sorted, zeted, peeled, and Iced
- 2 tsp. agave syrup
- 2 very thin slices red onion
- 1/8 tsp. salt
- 2 tbsp. Key lime juice
- 2 tbsp. olive oil
- Cayenne pepper, optional

Instructions:

Arrange watercress, avocado, onion, and oranges on two plates.

In a small bowl, combine lime juice, olive oil, agave syrup, salt, and cayenne pepper. Spoon dressing over salad when ready to serve.

Basil Avocado Pasta Salad

Bal leaves contain a variety of disease-fighting antioxidants, and they also treat tremors by serving as an adaptogen! Eat your greens and reap the benefits of basil in the delectable Bal Avocado Pasta Salad.

Ingredients:

- 1-pint cherry tomatoes halved
- 1 cup fresh basil, chopped
- 1 avocado, chopped
- 1/4 cup olive oil
- 1 tbsp. key lime juice
- 1 tsp. agave syrup
- 4 cups cooked spelled-pasta (you may substitute any type of spaghetti as long as it is authorised by Dr. Sebi's Cell Food Nutritional Guide)

Instructions:

- Place cooked pasta in a large bowl.
- Add avacado, bal, and tomatoe and stir until the ingredients are thoroughly mixed.
- In a small mixing bowl, combine the oil, lime juice, agave syrup, and ea alt. Pour over the pata and whisk to mix.

Wakame Salad

Sea veggies are high in antioxidants, fibre, and odne. This Wakame alad is a delicious and non-boring way to eat your greens!

Ingredients:

- 2 cup wakame tem (you can ue other ea vegetable a long a they appear on Dr. Seb' Nutrtonal Guide)
- 1 tbsp. agave syrup
- 1 tsp. onion powder
- 1 tbsp. key lime juice
- 1 tsp. ginger
- 1 tbsp. red bell pepper
- 1 tbsp. sesame oil
- 1 tbsp. sesame seeds

Instructions:

Soak wakame stems for 5-10 minutes and drain.

Combine eame ol, agave yrup, key lme juce, on powder, and gnger in a mixing bowl. Thoroughly whisk.

In a ervng pan, place wakame and bell pepper. Dressing should be poured on top.

Sprinkle with sesame seeds and enjoy!

The Grilled Romaine Lettuce Salad

Tired of the same old lettuce salad? This enticing recipe makes use of grilled romaine lettuce as a base.

Ingredients:

- 4 small heads romaine lettuce, rinsed
- Onion powder, to taste
- 1 tbsp. red onion, chopped finely
- 1 tbsp. key lime juice
- 4 tbsp. olive oil
- 1 tbsp. agave syrup
- 1 tbsp. fresh basil, chopped
- Sea salt and cayenne pepper, to taste

Instructions:

Place the lettuce, cut side down, in a large nonstick pan. Don't use any ol. Check the colour of the lettuce by turning it. Make sure the lettuce is browed on both sides.

Take the pan off the heat and allow lettuce to cool on a large platter.

In a small mixing bowl, combine red on with olve ol, agave yrup, key lme juce, and freh bal for the dreng. To taste, season with salt and cayenne pepper. Work well together.

Transfer the grilled lettuce to a serving dish and sprinkle with the dressing.

Enjoy!

Dandelion Strawberry Salad

Dandelion greens are used in traditional medicine to treat a variety of ailments. Recent research has proven that dandelon kills some bacteria and other germs and even has anti-cancer effects! Try them in a salad that combines sweet and salty ingredients for a delicious result!

Ingredients:

- 1 medium red onion, sliced
- 2 tbsp. grapeseed oil
- 4 cups dandelion greens
- 10 ripe strawberries, sliced
- Sea salt to taste
- 2 tbsp. key lime juice

Instructions:

Warm grappeeed ol over medium heat in a 12-inch nonstick fry pan. Add lced onon and a generous pinch of sea salt. Cook, stirring often, until onions are tender, softly brown, and reduced to approximately 1/3 of their original volume.

To strawberry lice wth 1 teapoon key lme juce in a tiny bowl. Wash the dandelon greens and chop them into bite-sized pieces if desired.

When the onions are nearly done, add the remaining key lime juice to the pan and continue cooking until it has thickened enough to coat the onions, perhaps a minute or two. Remove one from the heat.

In a salad bowl, combine the greens, onions, and strawberries with all their juices. Sprinkle with sea salt.

18. Pasta Salad

- 2 boxes of spelled penne

- 2 avocado chopped into tiny pieces

- 1/4 cup of almond milk

- 1/2 cup sun-dried tomatoes

- 1/2 cup of chopped onions

- 3-4 dashes of cilantro

- 1/4 cup of fresh lime juice

- 3 tbs of maple syrup

- 1/2 cup of olive oil

- 4 tbs of sea salt

Putting It All Together:

- Cook the pasta according to package directions.

- Combine everything in a large bowl.

- Toss until evenly distributed

Vegetable Salad

- 1/2 bunch watercress, torn
- (Remove ends and snap in half)
- 1/4 cup fresh lime juice
- 1/2 bunch romaine lettuce, torn
- 1/2 lb. fresh string beans
- 1/2 bunch cilantro, chopped fine
- 1/4 tsp. cumin
- 1/2 tsp. dill
- 1/2 cup olive oil
- Sweet basil to taste

Putting it all Together:

- Put olive oil in a bowl
- Marinade in refrigerator for 1-1/2 hours
- Add dill, cumin, basil, and lime juice
- Mix completely with lettuce, watercress, and cilantro.
- Enjoy!

Creamy Salad Dressing

- 2 green onions
- 4 tbs. almond butter
- 1/2 tsp. sweet basil
- 1/4 tsp. ground cumin
- 1 tsp. maple syrup
- 1/2 cup fresh lime juice
- 1/4 tsp. sea salt
- 1/4 tsp. thyme

Putting It All Together:

Add all ingredients and 2 tablepoon prng water to a gla bottle. Shake thoroughly and enjoy!

Vegetables:
20 Recipes

1. Roasted Tomato And Bell Pepper Soup

Ingredients:

- 3 sprigs fresh thyme

- 4 ripe Roma tomatoes

- Pure sea salt, to taste

- 3 red bell peppers

- 1/4 cup homemade vegetable broth with Dr. Sebi's approved vegetables

- Sesame oil

Putting It Together:

- Preheat oven to 375 degrees F.

- Chop peppers into quarters and remove centers.

- Slice the tomato and place it on an rmmed baking sheet alongside the bell peppers.

- Drizzle generously with sesame oil and sprinkle with sea salt.

- Scatter thyme over the vegetables.

- Roast in a preheated oven for 35-40 minutes.

- Transfer everything to a blender or food processor.

- Add warm broth and puree until smooth, adding more liquid as needed to get desired consistency.

- Add sea salt to taste. Pour into bowls and serve warm.

2. Chickpea Soup

Ingredients:

- 1 small zucchini
- 2 cups of chickpeas
- Water
- 1 bell pepper
- 1 small onion
- Seasoning of your choice

Instructions:

Put everything in a pot and cook on medium heat until the vegetables are aldente.

Once the oup and vegetable are ready, blend well using a multi-quick hand blender. It easiets that way and likes it. This will be plenty for several days.

3. Kale Soup

Ingredients:

- 5 cups vegetable broth
- 1 medium onion, chopped
- 1 medium chayote, diced
- 2 teaspoons dried sage
- 2 cups squash, diced
- 2 teaspoons dried thyme
- 3 cup kale, rinsed, tem removed, and very finely chopped
- Salt and pepper to taste

Instructions:

- Chop onions and let sit for 5 minutes.
- Heat 1 tablespoon broth in a medium soup pot.
- Cook the onion in the broth for about 5 minutes, stirring often.
- Add broth, chayote, and bring to a boil.
- When it reaches a boil, decrease the heat to a simmer and continue to cook for another 5 minutes. Cook until the squash is tender, about 15 minutes more.
- Cook for another 5 minutes after adding the greens and the rest of the ingredient. If you want to mmer for a longer period of time for more taste and rchne, you may need to add a little more broth.

4. Alkaline Electric Soup

- 1/2 lb. Garbanzo Beans (cooked)*
- 1-2 cups Kamut Pasta/Approved Pasta
- 1/2 cup Quinoa (Optional)
- 2 cups Mushrooms, chopped
- 1/2 cup of chopped Red Peppers
- 1 Zucchini Squash, chopped
- 2 cups Butternut Sq uash, chopped
- 1/2 cup of chopped Green Peppers
- 1 tablespoon of Grapeseed Oil
- 1 Small Red Onion, chopped
- 1 teaspoon dill
- 2 Roma Tomatoes, diced
- 1/2 gallon sprinkling water (adjust as needed)
- 1 teaspoon Red Cayenne Pepper
- 1 teaspoon Basil
- 1 teaspoon Oregano
- 1 tablespoon Sea Salt

Soak the garbanzo bean overnight and cook them before adding them to the Natve Stew.

Instructions:

- Pour the spring water into a large saucepan and heat over medium heat.
- Chop up all of your vegetables.
- Add the ingredient (including spices) to the pot and bring to a simmer for around 1 hour.
- Stir every 15 minutes.
- Enjoy!

5. Greens Soup Recipe

Ingredients:

- 1 bell pepper
- 2 cups leafy greens
- Water
- 1 small zucchini
- 1 small onion
- Seasoning of your choice

Instructions:

- Put everything in a pot and cook on medium heat until the vegetables are tender. Turn off the stove, allow it cool, and thoroughly combine.

6. Dr. Sebi's Cleansing Green Soup

The Cleaning Soup contains electric foods such as avocado and zucchini, as well as a high level of natural minerals. It also contains cleansing herbs that promote bowel motions and digestion while replenishing cellular nutrition.

Ingredients (Serves 4):

- 3 medium or 2 large yellow onions, peeled and coarsely chopped
- 1 bunch of dandelion greens
- 1 zucchini, washed but not skinned, roughly chopped
- 1/2 cup packed dill
- 1 bunch wild arugula
- 4 cup homemade vegetable broth (prepared only with approved vegetables)
- 1/4 avocado
- 1/2 cup packed basil
- 1/4 teaspoon sea salt
- Juice of 1 key lime
- 3 tablespoons grapeseed oil
- Cayenne pepper, to taste

Instructions:

To make the cleanng out, heat grapeed ol on a large pot over medum-hgh until warm.

Add onions and cook for 5 minutes, stirring occasionally, until translucent.

Cook for a further 5 minutes after adding the dandelon greens, zucchini, and wild arugula.

Pour in the homemade vegetable stock and bring to a boil, then reduce to a low heat and simmer, covered, for 15-20 minutes.

Let cool, uncovered, for 15 minutes.

Blend basil, avocado, dll, key lime juice, ea alt, and cayenne pepper in batches if required, until very smooth.'

7. Immunity-Boosting Soup

Comfort in a bowl! Enjoy the alkalne-electrc, nutrent-packed bowl of mmunty-bootng out!

Ingredients:

- 1 bell pepper
- 1/2 onion
- 1 cup mushrooms (any kind, except shiitake)
- 1 zucchini
- 1 tablespoon grapeseed oil
- 1 pack approved-flour noodle (pelled, amaranth, wild rice, etc.)
- Approved herbs
- 1 key lime
- 4 cups of water
- 1 cup cherry tomatoes
- Cayenne pepper with sea salt

Instructions:

- Cook the noodles following the package instructions.
- Chop the mushroom, bell pepper, and cherry tomatoes into tiny pieces. Sautee in the pan as well.
- Cut the onion into small chunks. Heat the grapeed ol and autée the on until transparent in a large pan.
- Grate the zucchini and add it to the pan.
- Add the water, sea salt, pepper, and spices. Bring to a boil over medium heat.
- Lower the heat after the boiling point has achieved. Cooked noodle should be added now. Allow me another 10 minutes.
- Adjust seasoning. Serve topped with more herbs and key lime juice.

8. Cucumber Basil Gazpacho

The Cucumber Basl Gazpacho is a creamy-tatng chlled out a natural for feeding an appetzer n little glae or a light lunch or supper on hot summer day.

Ingredients:

- 2 small handfuls fresh basil
- 1 perfectly ripe avocado
- 1 cucumber, seeded: kn left on, eed removed
- Juice of 1 key lime
- 2 cups of water
- 1 1/4 teaspoon sea salt

Instructions:

To prepare this chilled soup or "gazpacho". Refrigerate all ingredients until cold.

Place the chilled ingredient in a blender and blend until smooth, leaving a few flecks of green visible throughout.

Return to the refrigerator and chill until ready to serve.

Serve garnished with thinly sliced cucumber circles and basil leaves.

9. Veggie Fajitas Tacos

Do you want tacos? Consider the alkaline, plant-based option! The Mexican-inspired supper is a simple, tasty, and filling dish that comes together in less than 15 minutes!

Ingredients:

- 1 onion
- 2-3 large portobello mushrooms
- Juice of 1/2 key lime
- 2 bell peppers
- 6 corn-free tortillas (look for tortillas made with acceptable grains, such as these Kamut flour tortillas)
- 1 Tbsp. grapeseed oil
- Avocado
- Your preferred seasoning (onion powder, habanero pepper, cayenne pepper)

Instructions:

Remove the muhroom system, clean the gills if desired, and wet the top. Ice should be approximately 1/3 inch thick.

Thinly slice bell peppers and onion.

1 Tbsp. grapeseed oil, pepper, and onion in a large kettle over medium heat Cook for approximately 2 minutes.

Add the mushrooms and eaonng. Cook for another 7-8 minutes, or until well heated.

Warm the tortillas and ladle the fajita mixture into the centre of the tortillas. Serve with avacado and key lime juice.

10. Healthy "Fried-Rice"

You don't need Chinese takeout to fulfil your craving for fresh rice. Try the recipe instead!

Ingredients:

- 1/2 cup sliced bell peppers

- 1 cup cooked wild rice or quinoa

- 1 tbsp. grapeseed oil

- 1/2 cup sliced mushrooms

- 1/4 onion, cubed

- 1/2 cup sliced zucchini

- To taste, sea salt and cayenne pepper

Instructions:

Heat oil in a pan, and sautée onion until browned.

Cook for another 5 minutes after adding the remaining vegetables. Make sure they're not too clever.

Cook until just browned, then add the cup of boiled rice.

11. Lime And Olive Oil Dressing

- 1/2 cup olive oil

- 1/4 fresh lime, squeezed

- 1/4 tsp. sweet basil

- 1/8 cup spring water

- 1/4 tsp. thyme

- 1 tbs. maple syrup

- 1/4 tsp. ground cumin

- 1/4 tsp. oregano

Putting It All Together:

Put all ingredients in a glass bottle

Shake thoroughly and enjoy this delectable and simple salad dressing!

12. Fresh Tamarind Water

You may use the tamarnd paste from last week's recipe to make this wonderful "tamarnd water," which is ideal to accompany your fast.

Ingredients:

- 2 liters fresh spring water
- 100g tamarind pulp
- Agave syrup or date sugar
- 600ml boiling spring water

Instructions:

Pour boiling water over the tamarind pulp, and leave to soak for 20 minutes.

Break up the pulp with a fork and strain the mixture through a sieve into a basin. Using a poon, press as much pulp through as possible, and scrape any tamarnd puree from the bottom of the eve into the bowl.

Mix the resulting liquid with a liter of fresh spring water.

Sweeten with agave syrup or date sugar to taste.

13. All-Natural Tamarind Paste

The tamarind paste may be blended with water to make a refreshing drink or used as an ingredient in a dish to provide sweetness and flavour!

Ingredients:

- 3 cups of spring water
- 250 gr of natural tamarind

Instructions:

- Clean up the tamarnd. Check for any eed, skin, or unwanted particles and save them. Meanwhile, heat 2 cups of water.
- Soak the tamarind in 2 cups of boiling water for 45-60 minutes.
- Once the tamarind is soft, blend in a high-speed blender until very smooth.
- Using a sifter, sift the final mixture. Dcard any tone, eeed, or debr.
- Boil the resulting pulp for 5 minutes over medium flame.
- Once the paste has completely cooled, store it in an airtight container.

14. Dr. Sebi's "Heart-Friendly" Salsa

Now that you understand the importance of caring for your heart's health, it's time to try Dr. Sebi's "Heart-Friendly" Salasa! Dr. Seb's "Healthy" Salsa is spicy and delicious, packed with heart-healthy ingredients.

Ingredients:

- 2 tbsp. grapeseed oil

- 1 cup fresh blueberries

- 1/2 avocado, chopped

- 5 medium strawberries

- Juice of two key limes

- 1 pinch sea salt

- 1/3 cup chopped green bell pepper

- 1/4 red onion

Instructions:

- In a food processor or blender, combine blueberries, strawberries, onion, key lime zest, key lime juice, and green bell pepper and pulse 5-6 times.

- Scrape salsa into a bowl and fold in chopped avocado.

- Taste and seaon with sea salt and cayenne pepper if desired.

15. Dr. Sebi's Basil Pesto "Zoodles"

A light, healthful lunch made with fresh zucchini noodles, basil pesto, and cherry tomatoes. Make this meal for lunch or supper, or as a side dish!

Ingredients:

- 1/2 cup packed basil leaves
- 1 tbsp grapeseed oil
- 1/4 teaspoon Cayenne pepper
- 1 ripe avocado
- 1 lb zucchini, in small strips
- 1/4 cup walnuts
- 1/2 teaspoon sea salt
- 1/4 cup olive oil
- juice of one key lime
- 1 cup cherry tomatoes

Instructions:

- To make zoodles, start by sautéing zucchini noodles in grapeseed oil until soft but still crunchy.
- In a food processor or blender, combine the other ingredients and process into a creamy, thick paste.
- Add to the draned pata and to and combine. If you find the sauce too thick, add a splash of water.
- Serve with cherry tomatoes halves and decorate with shredded dissected coconut as "cheese".

16. Plant-Based Quinoa Bowl

This plant-based quinoa bowl is quick, filling, and delicious! The flavorful whole grain is ideal for quick lunches and dinners.

Ingredients:

- 1 tablespoon of grapeseed oil

- 1 cup cooked q uinoa

- 1 handful of approved greens

- 2 cups chopped approved vegetables, such as zucchini, cherry tomatoes, bell peppers, and so on

- Sea salt and cayenne pepper, to taste

Instructions:

- Heat a tablespoon grapeed ol in a big pan. Cook the chopped vegetables until soft.

- Combine the vegetables with the cooked unoa and fresh greens.

- Season with sea salt and cayenne pepper, to taste.

17. Alkaline Barb eq ue Sauce

- This recipe makes about 8-10 oz. of barbecue sauce.

- 6 Plum Tomatoes

- 2 tsp. Onion Powder

- 2 tbsp. Agave

- 1/4 cup White Onions, chopped

- 1/4 cup Date Sugar

- 1/4 tsp. Cayenne Powder

- 2 tsp. Smoked Sea Salt/Sea Salt

- 1/2 tsp. Ground Ginger

- 1/8 tsp. Cloves

- Hand Mixer

- Blender

Instructions

In a blender, combine all ingredients except the date sugar and blend until smooth.

Pour blended ingredients and date sugar into a saucepan at medium-high heat and stir occasionally until boiling.

Reduce heat to a simmer and cover for 15 minutes, stirring periodically.

Use a stick blender to make the sauce smoother.*

Cook for 10 minutes on low heat, or until the water evaporates.

Allow the sauce to cool and thicken more before serving.

Enjoy your Alkaline Barbecue Sauce!

18. Enoki And King Oyster Mushroom Soup

The muhroom serves a basic Asian tyle cuisine that will warm you up in the winter. It's tasty, filling, but best of all, it's quick and easy to make.

Ingredients

- Bell Peppers

- 1 King Oyster Mushroom

- 200g Watercress (or any greens you want)

- 1/4 pound Enoki Mushrooms

- 1 tbsp Grape Seed Oil

- Sea Salt (to taste)

- 4 tablespoons Irish Moss Gel (optional)

Instructions

- Wash all veggies and chop up the king oyster mushroom. You may cut crosswise into 2-inch chunks and then lengthwise.

- Separate the mushroom bundle into little bunches. These mushrooms grow tuck together, which is how they grow, so pull them apart into smaller bundles. There's no reason to segregate them all.

- Cut up the bell pepper and leafy greens into bite-size pieces.

- Bring a cup of spring water to a boil, then add 3-4 teaspoons of sea moss gel and stir it up. This makes the oup thcker.

- Once the water is boiling, decrease the heat to low and add the mushrooms and vegetables. Allow for a 5-minute simmer.

- Salt to taste and a tablespoon of grapeed oil

- 1 pkg. oyster mushrooms, sliced

- 3 tbs olive oil

- 2 zucchini, sliced

- 1 small red and green pepper, chopped

- 1/2 small yellow onion, chopped fine

- 1 cup broccoli, chopped fine

- 8 cherry tomatoes, chopped

Putting It All Together:

- Add tomatoes and onions

- Put olive oil in a heated stainless steel wok

- Add mushrooms and sauté another 3-4 min

- Add zucchini, bell peppers, broccoli and sauté 3-4 minutes

- 20. Cucumber Dressing

- Add your favorite seasonings and sauté 3-4 min

- 3 med. cucumbers, peeled

- 10 almonds, raw, unsalted

- 1/4 cup green onions, chopped fine

- 4 tbs. pure olive oil

- 1/2 tsp. thyme

- 1/4 cup fresh lime juice

- 1-1/2 cup spring water

- 1/2 tsp. sea salt

- 1/4 tsp. dill

- Few sprigs of cilantro, chopped

Putting It All Together:

Blend 10 almonds with spring water for 2 minutes on high speed.

Strain and set liquid aside

Cucumber purée in a blender with almonds

Add olive oil, lime juice, and remaining ingredients

Blend lightly, adding liquid as needed.

Pour over your salad and enjoy!

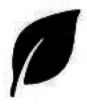

BOOK 9
Dr. Sebi's Recipes PART II

200 Delicious and Simple Recipes to Naturally Cleanse Your Liver, Lose Weight, and Lower High Blood Pressure, And Improve your health by detoxifying your body with an alkaline diet.

Dessert, Milk, Cheeses, And Snack: 30 Recipes

1. Irresistible Red Pepper Hummus

Hummus is the ultimate healthy snack to keep on hand. Chickpeas with red peppers are both nutritious and healthful. They have a high mineral, fibre, and antioxidant content.

Ingredients:

- 3 tablespoons homemade tahini

- 1 red bell pepper

- Sea salt and Cayenne pepper, to taste

- 1 cup cooked chickpeas (garbanzo beans)

- 2 tablespoons olive oil

- 2 tablespoons key lime juice

Instructions:

Place the red bell pepper on the stove burner and cook until the skin is browned. Remove from the heat and place in a plastic bag to cool for 10-15 minutes until they are cold enough to handle; then, remove the kn.

Combine the tahini and lime juice in a food processor bowl and process for 1 minute. Crape the edge and bottom of the bowl and process for 30 seconds longer. The extra time aids in "whipping" or "creaming" the tahn, making the hummu smooth and creamy.

Combine the olive ol, chickpea, sea salt, and cayenne pepper. Process for 30 seconds, scrape the side and bottom of the bowl, then process for another 30 seconds or until well blended.

This red pepper chckpea hummu would be a fantastic topping for the Plant-Based Quinoa Bowl.

2. Kamut Breakfast Porridge

With its nuttiness, Kamut, also known as Khoraan wheat, is a worthwhile addition to your diet. Kamut porridge is a filling, delectable breakfast packed with fibre and minerals such as magneum, elenum, manganee, and znc.

Ingredients:

- 1/2 teaspoon sea salt

- 4 tablespoons agave syrup

- 1 cup (7 ounces) Kamut

- 3/4 cup homemade walnut milk or off-jelly coconut milk

- 1 tablespoon coconut oil

Instructions:

- Mix the Kamut in a high-powered blender or food processor until you get about 1 1/4 cup of cracked Kamut.

- Mix cracked Kamut, walnut or coconut milk, and ea salt in a medium pot and stir to combine.

- Bring to a boil over high heat, then reduce to medium-low and simmer, stirring occasionally, for 10 minutes, or until thickened to your taste.

- Remove from heat and toss in the coconut oil and agave syrup. If desired, garnish with fresh fruit and enjoy your Kamut porridge!

3. Grilled Zucchini Hummus Wrap

This grilled zucchini hummus wrap is delicious and simple to make, making it excellent for lunch or dinner. This is the ideal quick and nutritious wrap recipes!

Ingredients:

- 1/4 sliced red onion

- 1 zucchini, ends removed and sliced

- 4 tbsp. homemade hummus (mashed garbanzo beans)

- 1 plum tomato, sliced, or cherry tomatoes, halved

- 1 cup romaine lettuce or wild arugula

- 1 tbsp. grapeseed oil

- 2 spelled flour tortillas
- Sea salt and cayenne pepper, to taste

Instructions:

Heat a skillet or grill to medium heat.

Toss sliced zucchini n grapeseed oil and sprinkle with sea salt and cayenne pepper.

Place toed, Iced zucchini straight on the grill and cook for 3 minutes, then turn and cook for another 2 minutes. Set zucchin aside.

Place the tortillas on the grill for about one minute, or until the grill marks are visible and the tortillas are ready.

Remove tortillas from grill and assemble with wrap, 2 tablepoon hummus, zucchini Ice, 1/2 cup green, onion, and tomato Ice.

Wrap tightly and enjoy it immediately.

4. Berry Sorbet

It's difficult to give up ice cream, but with the plant-baed, alkalne, healthy alternative, you won't have to! Dr. Seb' Berry Sorbet is the best tasting plant-based ice cream you've ever had.

Ingredients:

- 2 cups of water

- 1/2 cup date sugar

- 2 cups strawberries (pureed)

- 1/2 tsp. spelled flour

Instructions:

- Dissolve the date sugar and flour in the water in a large aucepan over low heat, then boil until thck, lke yrup, approximately ten minutes. Remove from the heat and allow to cool.

- When the syrup is completely cooled, add the pureed fruit and mix well.

- Cut the sorbet into chunks, then blend or mix in a food processor until smooth and creamy.

- Place in a plastic container and freeze uncovered until it is solid.

- Put the sorbet back into the freezer and allow to freeze for another 4 hours.

5. Zucchini Bread Pancakes

Ingredients:

- 2 cups spelled or Kamut flour
- 1 cup finely shredded zucchini
- 2 tbsp. date sugar
- 1 tbsp. grapeseed oil
- 1/4 cup mashed burro banana
- 1/2 cup chopped walnuts
- 2 cups homemade walnut milk

Instructions:

In a large bowl whisk flour and date sugar.

Pour in walnut milk and mashed burro banana Stir until just combined, being sure to cover the bottom of the bowl with a layer of dry mix. Stir in the shredded zucchini and walnuts.

Heat grapeseed oil in a griddle or skillet over medium-high heat.

Pour batter onto the griddle to make pancakes. Cook for 4 to 5 minutes on each side.

Serve with agave syrup and enjoy!

6. Juicy Portobello Burgers

The weather is heating up, so why not fire up the grill for these ncredble Jucy Portobello Muhroom Burgers? Make sure to serve these plant-based burgers on top of an approved-grain bun, such as Kamut, pelled, or unoa.

Ingredients:

- 2 large portobello mushroom caps
- 1 avocado sliced
- 1 tsp. dried oregano
- 3 tbsp. olive oil
- 1 cup purslane
- 2 tsp. dried basil
- 1 tomato sliced
- 1/2 tsp. Cayenne pepper

Instructions:

- Slice the mushroom tem and Ice about 1/2" of the mushroom top (as if slicing a bun).
- Mix olive oil, onion powder, bsail, oregano, and Cayenne pepper in a small bowl.
- Place the mushroom caps on a baking sheet with fol and a little grapeeed ol (to prevent sticking).
- Using a large spoon, marinade over each mushroom cap for around 10 minutes.
- Preheat the oven to 425°F and bake the mushrooms for about 10 minutes, checking the degree of readiness before flipping them to bake for another 10 minutes.
- Place the bottom of the mushroom cap on a plate, then add your topping of choice and top with the top portion of the baked mushroom cap.

7. Classic Homemade Hummus

The recipe for classic homemade hummus is a must-have for every home. The homemade hummus recipe is quick and easy to make, ultra-smooth and creamy, and tastes so fresh and tasty!

Ingredients:

- 2 tbsp. olive oil
- 1 cup cooked chickpeas
- A dash of onion powder
- 1/3 cup homemade tahini butter
- 2 tbsp. key lime juice
- Sea salt, to taste

Instructions:

- In a food processor or high-powered blender, combine all of the ingredients and serve.

8. Dr. Sebi's Fantastic Quinoa Bread

If you have a gluten allergy or intolerance yet miss bread, our unoa bread is for you! Dr. Seb's Fantatc Quinoa Bread is more than simply an alternative to wheat bread; it's also really good for you!

Ingredients:

- 300 g (10 ½ oz or 1 3/4 cups) whole uncooked quinoa seed
- 60 ml (2 fl oz / ¼ cup) grapeseed oil
- 1/2 cup water
- 1/2 key lime, juiced
- 1/2 teaspoon sea salt

Instructions:

Soak uinoa in plenty of cold water overnight in the fridge. Preheat the oven to 160 C / 320 F.

Dran the uinoa and rne well through an eve. Make sure the water is completely drained from your eve. Place the uinoa in a food processor.

Add ½ cup of water, grapeseed oil, sea salt, and key lime juice.

Mix for 3 minutes in a food processor. The bread mixture should approximate a batter consistency, with some whole quinoa remaining in the mix.

Spoon into a loaf tin lined with baking paper on all sides and the base.

Bake for 1 ½ hour until firm to touch and bounces back when pressed with your fingers.

Remove from the oven and cool for 30 minutes in the tn... then remove from the tn and cool thoroughly on a rack The bread should be light on the inside and crisp on the outside.

Cool completely before eating... and enjoy it!

9. Dr. Sebi's "Owl" Blueberry Pancakes

Now that you know that a plant-based diet is the greatest thing for your health and the planet, try Dr. Seb's Plant-Based "Owl" Blueberry Pancake! You won't be able to tell that these plant-baed Blueberry Pancake include no egg, milk, or butter. These pancake are incredibly thick, fluffy, and delicious, and your child will love the fun "owl" shape.

Ingredients:

- 1/4 cup homemade walnut milk
- 1/2 cup spelled, amaranth, or Kamut flour
- 1/3 cup blueberries
- 3 tbsp. date sugar
- 2 tbsp. grapeseed oil
- 1 pinch sea salt
- Agave syrup and extra fruit for serving

Instructions:

To make Dr. Sebi's plant-based "owl" blueberry pancake, start by whisking flour and date sugar together to get rid of any lumps. Pour homemade walnut mlk and grapeed ol into the flour/date sugar mxture and whisk until lumpy but mainly integrated with flour.

Add blueberries and fold in with a spatula to maintain lumps. DO NOT OVERMIX.

Preheat the griddle to 350°F (or a big pan to medium heat) and brush with a little layer of grapeed oil.

To the griddle, add 1/4-1/3 cup ervng of the pancake batter. Gently flatten with the back of a poon/ladle to the desired shape and to even out the batter.

Cook for about 2-3 minutes until the edges are slightly cooked and the bottom is golden.

Cook for another minute or two until the opposite side is golden.

To make the "owl" forms, serve with agave yrup and more fruit.

10. Scrumptious Mango "Cheesecake"

This scrumptious, plant-based mango "cheeecake" bursts with summer flavour. Creamy, rich, and packed of nutrients, this dessert will undoubtedly surprise your entire family!

Ingredients:

Crust:

- 1 cup dates
- 1/4 cup shredded dissected soft-jelly coconut
- 1 cup walnuts

Filling:

- 2 large mangos, peeled and cut into cubes
- 2 cups walnuts, soaked overnight & drained
- 1 cup homemade soft-jelly coconut milk
- 1/3 cup agave
- 1 tbsp. key lime zest
- Juice of 1 key lime
- 6 tbsp. coconut oil

Instructions:

Begin by lining an 8-inch baking sheet with parchment paper to prepare your plant-baed mango "cheesecake." Set aside.

Blend the walnuts, date, and hredded soft-jelly coconut until combined in a food processor or high-powered blender. If your dough isn't tacky enough, add a few more dates. Place the dough to the bottom of the pan and place it in the freezer.

Add the walnut and coconut milk to a food processor or high-speed blender. Blend for 2-3 minutes, or until perfectly smooth. Next, combine the coconut oil, agave syrup, key lime juice and zest, and mango cube. Blend until completely combined.

Pour the "cheesecake mixture into your pan, spreading evenly.

Place in the freezer for 2-4 hours before serving to firm up. Serve frozen, or thaw for 10-15 minutes for a softer texture.

11. Banana Nut Muffins

Now that you know all of the incredible benefits of banana, try this recipe for Banana Nut Muffins!

Ingredients:

- 1/4 cup grapeseed oil
- 1/2 cups approved-flour
- 3/4 cup date sugar
- 1/2 teaspoon sea salt
- 3/4 cup homemade walnut milk
- 2 medium ripe burro bananas, mashed
- 1/2 cup chopped walnuts, plus extra for sprinkling on top
- 1 medium ripe burro banana, cut into chunks
- 1 tablespoon key lime juice

Instructions:

To prepare your Banana Nut Muffins, begin by ṗ reheating your oven to 400F (200C). Lightly grease the cups of a muffin pan or fill with 12 non-stick liners.

In a large bowl, mix all of the dry ingredients.

Mix mashed banana with all of the wet ingredients in a medium bowl. Add the wet to the dry and stir until it just starts to come together. Take care not to go over mx. Add the chopped banana and walnuts and stir for 3 to 4 minutes.

Divide the batter evenly among the muffin pans and top with additional walnuts (optional). Bake for 22 to 26 minutes, or until the muffins have risen and are golden brown on the edges, and a toothpick inserted into the centre of a muffin comes out clean. Allow it cool for at least 10 minutes before enjoying.

12. Dr. Sebi's Portobello Mushroom Burgers

You're ready to taste Dr. Sebi's Portobello Mushroom Burger now that you know why you should wave meat goodbye! A delicious and simple marinade for these grilled plump portobello muhroom creates a burger that even a meat lover will like!

Ingredients:

- 2 tbsp agave syrup

- 6 large portobello mushroom caps

- 2 tbsp key lime juice

- 4 tbsp avocado oil

- Sea salt and Cayenne pepper to taste

- Extra veggies: bell peppers, onions, mushrooms, etc.

Instructions:

To prepare Dr. Sebi's Portobello Muhroom Burgers, begin by combining the prepared ingredients in a small bowl.

Pour the marnade over the top of the mushroom cap cap de in a 913 baking dish. Allow the mushrooms to soak in the marinade for about 30 minutes, periodically bruhing the top of the mushrooms.

Grill mushroom for 5-7 minutes per side, starting with the cap side down. Continue to bruh the muhroom with the marinade as they cook.

Serve on toasted (approved-grain) bread with your favourite toppings or with mixed vegetables.

13. Dr. Sebi's Fat-Free Peach Muffins

Are you concerned about the health of your gallbladder? A low-fat diet can help manage and reduce gallstone symptoms. This recipe for Dr. Sebi's Fat-Free Muffin is delicious, fat-free, and packed with good-for-you ngredent.

Ingredients:

- 2 tablespoons warm spring water
- 1 tablespoon agave syrup
- 1/2 teaspoon mashed burro banana
- 2 large peaches about 2 cups, chopped
- 1/4 cups homemade walnut milk
- 2 teaspoons key lime juice
- 1/2 cup date sugar
- 2 tablespoons chopped walnuts
- 1/4 teaspoon salt
- 2 cups spelled flour

Instructions:

Preheat oven to 400 F. Prepares your muffin pan by oiling it with a little grapeseed oil.

Peel the peach (if they are extremely ripe, the skin may easily peel off; if not, put them in boiling water for 30 seconds and allow to cool before peeling) and remove the pit. Chop into 1/2-inch pieces. Combine with agave syrup (optional) and set aside.

Add the key lime juice and walnut milk to the mashed burro banana and combine well.

In a large bowl, combine the flour, sea salt, and date sugar. Mix well.

Add the liquid ngredent and tr only until combined; the batter will be thck. Fill in the peaches, making sure they're evenly distributed throughout the batter.

Fill each muffin cuup to within 1/2-inch of the top. Smooth the top of each muffin and, if desired, top with chopped walnuts.

Bake for 15-20 minutes, or until a toothpick comes out clean. Allow the muffn to cool before serving.

14. Dr. Sebi's Raw Energy Balls

Simple, easy, raw, alkaline-electronic nack to provide you with tonnes of energy and nourishment in just one bite!

Ingredients:

- 1/2 cup blueberries or other approved fruit you prefer
- 1 tablespoon agave syrup
- 1/2 cup dried dates
- 2 cups shredded soft-jelly coconut
- 1 tsp. date sugar
- 1/2 cup walnuts or Brazil nuts
- Pinch of sea salt

Instructions:

- Begin by proceeng the walnut n a food proceor or high-peed blender or Brazil nuts till you get a fne powder to make Dr. Sebi's raw energy balls.
- Add the dried date, ugar date, and blueberre. Pour the agave slowly until you have a smooth surface.
- Chill mixture for 30 min- 2 hours.
- Roll into 1 tablespoon balls and roll in more shredded coconut if desired. You may keep it in the fridge for up to a week or in the freezer for up to three months.

15. Dr. Sebi's Magic Green Falafels

You'll like Dr. Sebi's Magic Green Flaafel Recipe! It is quick and simple to prepare, extremely flavorful, alkaline-free, and requires no frying.

Ingredients:

- 1/3 cup red bell pepper, chopped
- 2 cups dry garbanzo beans (chickpeas)
- 1/2 cup fresh dill
- 1 large onion, chopped
- 1/4 tsp. oregano
- 1/2 cup garbanzo bean flour
- 2/3 cup fresh basil
- 1 tsp. sea salt
- Grapeseed or avocado oil for frying

Instructions:

To make your Magic Green Falafels, begin by cooking the chickpeas until soft. Drain and rinse the beans.

Place the chickpeas in a food processor with all of the other ingredients: onion, red bell pepper, fresh herbs, sea salt, oregano, and flour.

Pulse until all of the ingredients are finely chopped and a coarse meal form. Scrape down the edge and pulse again until the texture resembles a fine meal. Taste and adjust the amount if necessary.

Transfer the mixture to a large mixing basin. Form little balls or thick discs with your hands and place them on a lined baking sheet. Chill for at least 1 hour in the refrigerator.

Fill a large skillet with oil to a depth of about 1 inch. Heat for 5-7 minutes on medium heat. When the oil is hot, fry the Magic Green Falafels for 2-3 minutes per side.

16. Dr. Sebi's Alkaline-Electric Spelt Meal Raisin Cookies

Now that you know everything there is to know about the amazing nutritional benefits of raisins, you must try Dr. Sebi's Alkaline-Electric Splt Meal Raisin Cooke! They are a delightful, healthful snack that both kids and adults will enjoy.

Ingredients:

- 2/3 cups homemade applesauce (pureed apple)
- 3 cups spelled flour
- 1/3 cup agave syrup
- 1 1/2 cups dates, pitted
- 1/2 teaspoon sea salt
- 2 tablespoons water
- 1/3 cup grapeseed oil
- 1 cup raisins

Instructions:

- To make your alkalne-electrc spelled meal ran cookies, begin by blending the pelled meal flour, date, and sea salt in a food processor until well combined.
- Transfer to a bowl; add remaining ingredients and mix.
- Roll a pound of cooked dough into a ball and lay it on a baking sheet lined with parchment paper. Flatter with your fingers or a fork.
- Preheat the oven to 350°F for 18-20 minutes. Allow to cool before enjoying your alkaline-electric pelled meal rain cookies!

17. Dr. Sebi's No-Bake Energy Balls

The BEST No-BAKE Energy Ball Recept! Easy to make, great for a healthy snack or breakfast, and kids adore these!

Ingredients:

- 1 cup walnuts
- 3/4 cup raspberries
- 2 2/3 cup shredded soft-jelly coconut meat
- 10 dates
- 1 pinch sea salt

Instructions:

- To prepare Dr. Seb's No-Bake Energy Balls, combine all ingredients in a food processor or blender. Process or blend until all of the ingredients are combined.
- Use moist hands to form the no-bake energy balls.
- When all balls have been formed, place the tray in the freezer 20-30 minutes.
- Enjoy!

18. Fruity Smoothie Bowl

Make a delicious breakfast dish with your favourite fruits. The fruity moothe bowl is filled with nutrients and taste!

Ingredients:

- 1/4 cup blueberries

- 1/4 cup seeded grapes

- 1 cup mixed berries

- 1 burro banana

- 1 tablespoon of your preferred nut butter (homemade tahini, or homemade walnut or Brazil nut butter)

- 2 – 3 tablespoons walnut or soft-jelly coconut milk

- 1 mango

- 1/4 cup strawberries

- Date sugar or agave syrup, to taste

Instructions:

- Add the berries and burro banana to a blender and mix on low until smooth.

- Add a bit of soft-jelly coconut milk or homemade walnut milk, nut butter, and date ugar or agave syrup (optional), and blend on low until the mixture reaches a creamy consistency.

- Scoop into a bowl and top with the rest of the fruit: blueberries, grapefruit, mango, and strawberries.

19. Green Pancakes

Are you concerned about muscle loss or obtaining enough protein on a plant-based diet? Don't be concerned! Chickpea (garbanzo bean) flour, the main ingredient in Dr. Sebi's Green Pancake, is naturally rich in protein and fibre.

Ingredients:

- 1/2 cup fresh spring water
- 1 tablespoon agave syrup
- 1/2 teaspoon sea salt
- 1/2 cup chickpea flour
- 1 handful amaranth greens
- 1/4 cup blueberries
- 1 burro banana
- 1 tablespoon of your preferred nut butter (homemade tahini, or homemade walnut or Brazil nut butter)

Instructions:

In a blender, combine all of the ingredients and mix until smooth. Be careful not to add too much water or they will not fluff or cook as well.

Allow the batter to sit for 5-10 minutes. While it's resting, heat a nonstick frying pan over medium-high heat.

Scoop the batter into the pan to make 6 tiny pancakes. If you like, you may adjust the size to make 3 giant pancakes, 4-5 medium pancakes, or 6 little pancakes.

Allow them to cook until there are some bubbles in the batter and they begin to look fluffy and cooked around the edges. Fluff and heat for another couple of minutes.

Serve decorated with blueberries, burro banana, and agave syrup. Enjoy your Green Pancakes!

20. Alkaline-Electric Classic Apple Bake

This simple recipe for classic baked apples is loaded with fresh, sweet, and tart apples with a hearty dose of pce. Enjoy the healthy, alkaline-electric version of the classic apple bake.

Ingredients:

- 3 to 4 Gala or Honeycrisp apples, depending on size (Read about our app selection here)

- 1 tablespoon chopped walnuts

- 3 tablespoons agave syrup
- Pinch of cloves

Instructions:

Begin by preheating the oven to 350°F for this classic apple bake. Only choose and apply. Place in a large bowl and drizzle with agave syrup. Str well to coat thoroughly.

Combne clove and walnut and prnkle over agave-coated apple, stirring constantly to coat. Allow around 5 minutes to encourage the juice to flow out.

Arrange sliced apples into a casserole dish.

Bake for 15 minutes, then cover with foil and bake for another 35-40 minutes, or until the apples are bubbly and your house smells amazing!

21. Plant-Based Chickpea Quinoa Burgers

Who says you can't enjoy burgers on a plant-based diet?

Ingredients:

- 1 1/2 cups cooked quinoa

- 1/4 chopped onion

- 2 tablespoons fresh (approved) herbs of your choice

- 1 1/2 cup cooked chickpeas (garbanzo beans)

- 2 tablespoons water

- 1/4 cup cooked amaranth

- 1 tablespoon per patty of raw homemade sesame "tahini" butter

- Sea salt and cayenne pepper, to taste

- Vegetables of your choice for ervng: cherry tomatoes, green (recommended) lettuce such as wild arugula, watercress, or lettuce, etc.

Instructions:

Preheat the oven to 375 degrees F.

In a food processor, combine the onion and herbs. Pule until they are finely chopped. Continue to pule after adding your chickpeas, unoa, and amaranth. Don't purée the mixture; you want it to be a little chunky.

Add sea salt and cayenne pepper and process until a dough forms. While the food processor is operating, add water and the dough will come together. The mixture should be thick, not runny or dry. Place the bowl in the refrigerator for 15 minutes to cool.

Once chilled, separate the mixture into 8 eq ual-sized patties.

Place your patte on a baking sheet lined with parchment paper and bake for 20 minutes. Finish with a brisk 2 - 3-minute brol to get the patties nice and browned.

Serve on a certified-flour bun with handmade raw sesame "tahn" butter and wild arugula, watercress, or lettuce.

22. Tef Grain Burgers

These Tef Grain Burger demonstrate that plant-based food may be both healthy and delicious! Your family will enjoy this plant-based dessert!

Ingredients:

- 1 1/2 cups garbanzo bean (chickpea) flour
- 1 1/2 cups cooked tef grain
- 1/4 of an onion,
- Diced 1 teaspoon basil
- 1/4 cup bell peppers, finely diced
- 1 tablespoon grapeseed oil
- 1 teaspoon dill
- 1 teaspoon oregano
- Sea salt and cayenne pepper, to taste

Instructions:

- Pour a tablespoon of grapeseed oil and auteé onon into a pan and tender until they are tender.
- In a large mixing bowl, combine the cooked vegetables with the remaining ingredients.
- Form patties using your hands and cook in a kllet for about 3 minutes on each side, or until crispy. Enjoy!

23. Alkaline-Electric Ice Cream

Satisfy your cravings for ice-cream with only alkaline-electric, good-for-you ingredients.

Ingredients:

- 2 ripe mangoes

- Agave syrup or date sugar (optional).

- 3 tablespoons of homemade walnut milk

- 2 burro bananas

Instructions:

Peel and cut the mangoes into cubes. Peel the burro bananas as well, and slice.

Place the mango and banana chunks on a baking sheet lined with parchment paper. Freeze.

Place your frozen fruit in the bowl of a food processor or strong blender. Add the homemade walnut milk and any sweetener.

Blend for around 3 - 4 minutes. It will appear that it will never become ice cream-like, but persevere. You may need to top through to puh it down the de and tr t around a bt.

24. Alkaline Electric Flatbread

This recipe makes 4 – 6 servings.

- 1 tbsp. Sea Salt

- 2 cups Spelt Flour

- 2 tsp. Onion Powder

- 2 tbsp. Grapeseed Oil

- 3/4 cup Spring Water

- 2 tsp. Oregano

- 2 tsp. Basil

- 1/4 tsp. Cayenne

The best part about this recipe is that you can make it in about 20 minutes and it's great for andwche, wrap, or tiny pizza.

Instructions:

- Mix flour and seasonings until well blended.

- Blend with an oil and around 1/2 cup of water. Mix with water slowly until it forms a ball.

- Add flour to the work surface and knead the dough for about 5 minutes, then divide the dough into 6 equal halves.

- Roll out each ball into about 4-inch circles.

- Place in a nonstick skillet over medium-high heat, flipping every 2-3 minutes until done.

- Enjoy your Alkaline Flatbread!

25. Vegan Flatbread Pizza

Ingredients

- Onion Powder
- Green / Red Bell Pepper
- Red / White Onions
- Roma Tomatoes
- Agave Nectar
- Mushrooms
- Spelled Flour
- Avocado
- Oregano
- Grapeseed Oil
- Sea Salt
- Food Processor or Blender
- Brazil Nut Cheese
- Alkaline Pizza Crust

Measurements:

- 1 tsp. Oregano
- 1 1/2 cups Spelt Flour
- 2 tsp. Agave
- 1 tsp. Onion powder
- 2 tsp. Sesame seeds
- 1 tsp. Sea Salt
- 1 cup Spring Water
- 2 tsp. Grapeseed Oil

Instructions:

- Preheat the oven to 400°F.

- In a medium-sized bowl, combine all of the ingredients, adding only 1/2 cup of boiling water. Slowly add water until the dough forms a ball; if too much water is used, add more flour.

- Coat your baking sheet lightly with grape eed ol, add flour to your hands, and roll out the dough onto the baking sheet.

- Bruh the top of the crust with grape eed oil and poke a hole in it with a fork. Bake the crust for around 10-15 minutes.

- Prepare your tomato or avocado pizza sauce while the crust is baking. (Recipes Below)

- Once the crust is done, top with your pizza sauce, Brazil nut cheese*, muhroom, peppers, and onions. Bake the pizza for around 15-20 minutes.

- Enjoy your Alkaline Veggie Pizza!

- The nut cheese helps to cook the toppings while baking; if you don't have any nut cheese, I recommend lightly sauteing the toppings before baking.

26. Irish Moss Papaya Jelly

This is a simple and delicious recipe for papaya jelly that combines papaya with our Irh mo gel.

Ingredients

- 3 tablespoon Irish Moss Gel
- 1 Papaya
- 1-2 handful of Strawberries

Instructions:

- Remove the eed by cutting up the papya. Scoop out the papaya fruit and place it in the blender.

- Add Irish mo gel and any desired fruit for sweetness (which papaya frequently loses when combined with Irh mo). Remember that fruit with a high water content may require more Irish mo to firm up, so just use a few (5 or 6 strawberries). Optionally, add star anise.

- Blend for 1-2 minutes, or until smooth. Tate the mixture to check for desired sweetness. Because of the tate-texture relationship, the taste will be somewhat different once it becomes firm.

- Pour the mixture into a container, cover, and refrigerate overnight. Because of the Irish mogel, the mixture should be firm like jelly by morning.

27. Banana Nut Vegan Ice Cream

This is a wonderful homemade banana vegan ice cream that can be created with a few simple ingredients and uses coconut jelly and Irh mo gel as a thickener.

Ingredients

- 3 tbsp Irish Moss Gel
- 5 Burro Bananas
- 7 Walnuts
- Coconut Jelly
- Date Sugar (optional)

Instructions:

Soak the nut for a few hours or overnight, then strain and remove any flaky skin for a smoother texture.

Scoop out your soft coconut jelly from a fresh coconut and place it in a blender; mix until smooth.

Peel the bananas and place them in a blender. Blend until smooth with the coconut jelly.

Add 3-5 tablespoons of Irish moss gel then blend until smooth.

Add a dash of date sugar to sweeten if you like and blend.

Pour the mixture into a bowl for storing, then drain the water from the walnuts and chop into small pieces. The size of the pebbles should be fine. They should be able to cut rather easily after being moistened.

Pour the walnut pieces into your cream cheese mixture and whisk to evenly distribute the nuts. To level the surface of the mixture, use the back of a spoon.

Cover and place in the freezer for 4 to 6 hours. If you freeze it for too long, it will become too hard. If you put it in for too long, just take it out and let it defrost for a while before eating. It can also be refrigerated or consumed at room temperature. It's incredibly sweet, and the walnut adds a nice crunch.

28. Walnut Milk

Walnut milk is simple to make, but it takes some time to prepare since the nuts must be soaked overnight. Here's a simple recipe; feel free to adjust the numbers if you want to create more, i.e. 200g walnuts to 1.5 litres (1.5 quarts) water.

Ingredients

- 750ml spring water
- 100g walnuts

Instructions:

- Strain and sq ueeze with a nut milk bag.
- Add to blender with water (750ml) and blend.
- Rinse the nuts.
- Place in the fridge to chill.
- Soak nuts in water overnight.

29. Bromide Hemp Seed Milk

Combine Dr. Seb's bromide powder with hemp milk to create a great and healthy drink with anti-inflammation properties. You will undoubtedly suffer from ad if you suffer from bad breath, pulmonary diseases, repratory ue, or dyentery. If you've used Dr. Seb's Bromide Plu Powder, you'll know that it can have an unpleasant odour or aftertaste. The active ingredient, Bladderwrack (a kind of eaweed), gives it a fishy or oceanic odour. The recipe was created to make it taste even better.

Ingredients

- 1 tbsp Bromide Powder
- 3 cups Water
- Dates (about 4)
- 2 tbsp Hemp Seeds

Instructions:

Rinse the hemp seed and mix with 2-3 cups of water (hot or cold) until fully combined. This will provide you with hemp seed milk.

Remove the eed off your date and place it in a container. Use more date for a sweeter taste. If you have a weet tooth, I recommend using 6. However, if you choose, you may leave the date out.

Stran the hemp eed mlk into a container and write the date on it. This will allow you to combine your dates a bit earlier.

Make sure to clean the grt and other residue out of your blender since you'll most likely be left with a piece of hemp eed at the bottom t - wash them out and wash your traner.

Return the hemp seed milk and date to the blender and pulse a few times to chop the date. Then use your blender to smooth everything up.

If desired, add 1-2 tablespoons of Dr. Seb's Bromde Plus and a dash of tar ane. Continue mixing for 30 seconds to a minute more.

Serve your delicious drink and enjoy hot or cold.

30. Vegan Nut Cheese

The texture of this vegan cheese is similar to rcotta but significantly firmer, even keeping the form of the container it's made in. It may also be used as a cheese spread and to make delicious hummus. The walnut cheese has a gritty texture and a darker colour, but it still has a nice flavour and can be stored in the refrigerator for 5 to 7 days. It may also be frozen and preserved for a month or longer.

Ingredients

- 1 tsp Coconut Oil

- 100g Walnuts

- 2 tbsp Tahini Sesame Paste

- Springwater

- 2 tsp Sea Salt (to taste)

- 3 tbsp Irish Moss Gel

Instructions:

- Soak the nuts overnight, strain, and remove any flaky skins for a smoother texture.

- Place nuts in a blender, beginning with an uarter cup of water. Keep a cup of water nearby so that you may add more while combining. Pulse the nut first, then blend it, slowly adding water as needed until you get a creamy l sould. It should have the consistency of a Ranch alad dressing or something like.

- Blend in 3 tablespoons Irish mo gel until smooth. You should notice a slight change in texture.

- Add 2 tablespoons of sesame paste, 1/2 tablespoon of coconut oil (optional), and a teaspoon of salt. Blend and mix well.

- Taste the mixture and season with extra salt if necessary. The eame paste and salt give it a cheesy flavour.

- Once you've found the taste you're looking for, Pour the mixture into a jar and seal it. Place it in the refrigerator to chill. It should harden up after a few hours or by the next day. If you're gentle enough with it, you might even be able to Ice it.

Herbal Tea Recipes:
35 Recipes

1. Dr. Sebi Herbal Smoothie

The use of herb to eliminate pathogens was first documented over 4,000 years ago. Dr. Seb uses ancient healing methods in modern times, such as this delectable Herbal Smoothe.

Ingredients:

- 1 burro banana
- Your favorite Dr. Sebi's Herbal Tea
- 1 tablespoon date sugar or agave syrup
- 1 tablespoon walnuts

Instructions:

- To make Dr. Seb' Herbal Smoother, begin by preparing your Dr. Seb' Herbal. Tea according per the package directions.
- Let coolTo make Dr. Seb' Herbal Smoother, begin by preparing your Dr. Seb' Herbal. Tea according per the package directions. Let cool
- Enjoy!

2. Mood-Boosting Smoothie

This Mood-Inducing Smoothe has all of the components needed to boost your mood and get you ready for a good day! The berries reduce inflammation, while the healthy fats from the coconut fuel your baby.

Ingredients:

- 1/2 cup soft-jelly coconut meat
- 1 cup of Dr. Sebi's Nerve/Stress Relief Herbal Tea.
- Date sugar or agave syrup, to taste.
- 1 cup strawberries

Instructions:

- To make the Mood-boosting Smoothie, start with one cup of dtlled water and add 1/2 tablespoon of Dr. Seb' Nerve/Stre Relef Herbal Tea. Tran tran tran tran tran tran tran tran tran Let cool.
- Blend the tea with the rest of the ingredients in a high-speed blender.
- Enjoy!

3. Dr. Sebi's Energy-Boosting Green Smoothie

Do you believe you could get up in the morning without coffee? Read our most recent article to discover a natural way to get a boost of energy without caffeine, while sipping on Dr. Sebi's Energy-Boosting Green Smoothie!

Ingredients:

- 2 handfuls of greens (dandelion greens, amaranth greens, lettuce, or wild arugula)
- 1/2 tsp. Bromide Plus Powder
- 1/2 seeded cucumber
- 1 burro banana
- 1 apple
- 1 cup soft-jelly coconut milk
- 1 tablespoon walnuts

Instructions:

- Begin by combining all ngredent in a high-peed proceor to make your energy-bootng green moothe.
- Serve on a tall glass, and enjoy!

4. Dr. Sebi's Anti-Bloat Smoothie

There are several natural ways to combat belly bloat, such as drinking a green smoothie chock full of anti-bloat ngredent to feel better.

Ingredients:

- 1/2 teaspoon Bromide Plus Powder
- 1/2 cup soft-jelly coconut water
- 1/2 cucumber, seeded
- 1/2 cup Dr. Sebi's Stomach Relief Herbal Tea
- 1 burro banana

Instructions:

- Prepare the tea and let cool.
- Blend all the ingredients in a high-speed blender and enjoy.

This anti-bloat moothe will assist you in fighting stomach bloat the proper way. While the other anti-bloat ingredients work, the tea will relax your stomach and provide quick comfort. Cucumbers are high in water, which helps you stay hydrated, but banana and coconut water are high in potassium, which aids in water retention. The Bromide Plu Powder will give your anti-bloat smoothie the boost it needs to energise you and keep your stomach and digestion working properly.

5. Dr. Sebi's Relaxation Smoothie

When left untreated, tre can contribute to a variety of health problems. What can you do to keep your stress to a minimum? While you p th delcou Relaxation Smoothe, read our post on tp for treng le! With hydrating cantaloupe, zucchini, and coconut water, this calming elixir is the ideal drink to unwind after a hard day.

Ingredients:

- 1/2 burro banana
- 1 cup cantaloupe
- 1/2 cup Dr. Sebi's Nerve/Stress Relief Herbal Tea
- 1 zucchini, chopped
- 1/2 cup soft-jelly coconut water

Instructions:

- To make your Relaxation Smoothie, first prepare the tea according to package directions and set aside to cool.
- Blend all the ingredients, including the tea, in a high-speed blender.
- Pour in a cup and enjoy!

6. Dr. Sebi's Watermelon Refresher

The Watermelon Refresher: a delicious drink full of natural electrolytes and antioxidants!

Ingredients:

- Zest and juice of 1 key lime
- 4 cups cubed watermelon
- Date sugar, to taste
- 2 cups soft-jelly coconut water

Instructions:

- Place the watermelon, lime juice, and zest in a blender or food processor and blend until smooth.
- Adjust the sweetness of the mixture with the date ugar. Keep in mind that the taste will be watered down once you add the soft-jelly coconut water.
- Serve 2/3 watermelon mxture and 1/3 oft-jelly coconut water on a tall gla. Mix with a spoon and enjoy your Watermelon Refreher!

7. Fruity Smoothie Bowl

Make your favourite fruit into a delectable breakfast dish. The delicious moothe bowl is high in nutrients and flavour!

Ingredients:

- 1/4 cup seeded grapes

- 1 cup mixed berries

- 1/4 cup strawberries

- 1 burro banana

- 1 tablespoon of your preferred nut butter (homemade tahini, or homemade walnut or Brazil nut butter)

- 1/4 cup blueberries

- 2 – 3 tablespoons walnut or soft-jelly coconut milk

- 1 mango

- Date sugar or agave syrup, to taste

Instructions:

- Add the berries and the burro banana to a blender and blend on low until small bits remain.

- Add a touch of soft-jelly coconut or homemade walnut milk, nut butter, and date ugar or agave yrup (optional), and blend on low until the mixture reaches a soft-serve consistency.

- Scoop into a bowl and top with the rest of the fruit: blueberries, grapes, mango, and strawberries.

8. Magnesium-Boosting Smoothie

Did you read the article on why magneum is so important? Go read it to discover out, and then come back to try the smoothe! This creamy, crumbly concoction is a delectable way to add magnesium to your diet.

Ingredients:

- 1/2 burro banana

- 1 cup fresh spring water

- 2 strawberries

- 1/4 cup Brazil Nuts

- 1/2 cup figs

Instructions:

- Blend all ingredients in a high-speed blender.

- Add more water if the mixture is too thick

- Enjoy!

If you want to boost the Magneum content of this moothe, add a teapot of Dr. Seb's Bromde Plus Powder. All of Dr. Sebi's Cell Food products include the highest concentration of Magnesium. Bromide Plus Powder acts as a natural diuretic; it improves appetite, regulates bowel movements, and aids in overall digestion.

9. Sugar Detox Smoothie

Drinking green can help reduce ugar cravng, especially if you have it on an empty stomach. Try the amazing Sugar Detox Smoothie for breakfast and let us know how you felt.

Ingredients:

- 1 squeeze of key lime

- 1/2 avocado

- 1 handful of "approved" greens, such as callaloo, watercress, or dandelion greens

- 1 cup homemade soft-jelly coconut milk

- 1 teaspoon of Dr. Sebi's Bromide Plus Powder

Instructions:

- Blend all ingredients in a high-speed blender until creamy. Enjoy!

10. Dr. Sebi's Immunity-Boosting Smoothie

Give your immune system a much-needed vitamin boost with this antioxidant-packed concoction: Dr. Sebi's Immunity Boosting Smoothe

Ingredients:

- 1 cup brewed Dr. Sebi's Immune Support Herbal Tea
- 1/2 mango
- 1 tablespoon date sugar or agave syrup
- 1 Seville orange
- 1 key lime, juiced
- 1 tablespoon coconut oil

Instructions:

- Boil two cups of purified water and add one and a half tablespoons of Dr. Seb's Immune Support Herbal Tea. Simmer for around 15 minutes. Allow to cool before using, tran.
- Peel the Seville orange and cut the mango into chunks.
- Blend all the ingredients in a high-speed blender. Enjoy!

11. Heart-Healthy Smoothie

In addition to the heart-healthy fat from the nut, this apple smoothie has cholesterol-lowering soluble fibre from the apple and walnut milk, as well as antioxidants from the blueberries.

Ingredients:

- 1 cup homemade walnut milk
- 1 Braeburn apple, or another kind of organic apple
- 1 cup blueberries
- 1/4 cup of Brazil nuts
- 1/2 tablespoon of date sugar or agave syrup
- 1 cup of approved greens (dandelion greens, turnip greens, watercress, etc.)

Instructions:

- Blend all the ingredients in a high-speed blender and enjoy!

12. Hormone-Balancing Smoothie

The smoothie is a terrific way to start your day, invigorate you, and naturally balance your hormones to set you up for success in living your most vibrant life.

Ingredients:

- 1/4 large avocado
- 1 1/4 cup homemade walnut milk
- 3 tablespoons hemp seeds
- 2 handfuls of dandelion greens
- 1/3 cup diced zucchini

Instructions:

- Blend all the ingredients in a high-speed blender and enjoy!

13. The Kidney Cleanse Juice

Detoxify and cleanse your kidney and urinary system with this extremely potent drink. The Kidney Cleanse Juice for You!

Ingredients:

- 2-3 key limes
- 1-2 cups of soft-jelly coconut water
- 1/2 tsp. Bromide Plus Powder
- 1 bunch basil or sweet basil leaves
- 4 seeded cucumbers

Instructions:

- Cucumber, basil, and key lime juice If you don't have a juicer, blend them in a high-speed blender with the soft-jelly coconut water.
- Pour the juice into a large glass and top with the soft-jelly coconut water and Bromde Plu Powder. Mx well and have fun!

14. Super Hydration Smoothie

With this "super hydration smoothie," you can avoid dehydration. Watermelon, cucumber, and raspberries all have a high-water content, are low in sugar, and strong in minerals and antioxidants. And they're all refrehing!

Ingredients:

- 1/4 seeded cucumber
- 1 cup watermelon
- 1/2 cup raspberries
- 1/2 cup soft-jelly coconut water
- 1 key lime, juiced

Instructions:

- To prepare the "super hydraton," smoothe, peel, and core the cucumber, then cut into tiny chunks.
- Blend all ingredients in a high-speed blender.
- Refrigerate until you are ready to drink. Enjoy!

15. Immunity-Boosting Smoothie

Boost your immune system with this refreshing mango-orange smoothie.

Ingredients:

- 1 cup brewed Dr. Sebi's Immune Support Herbal Tea
- 1/2 mango
- 1 tablespoon date sugar or agave syrup
- 1 Seville orange
- 1 key lime, juiced
- 1 tablespoon coconut oil

Instructions:

- 2 cups pure water + 1 12 teaspoon Dr. Sebi's Immune Support Herbal Tea Cook for around 15 minutes. Allow to cool, train.
- Peel the Seville orange and cut the mango into chunks.
- Blend all the ingredients in a high-speed blender. Enjoy!

16. Creamy Relaxing Smoothie

The avocados and bananas in the smoothie are great for lowering blood pressure, which can help you relax. Packed with healthy fats from avacado and banana, this anti-tre moothe will keep you feeling fuller for longer, preventing mood swings.

Ingredients:

- 1/4 seeded cucumber

- 1/2 cup prepared Dr. Sebi's Nerve/Stress Relief Herbal Tea

- 1 cup soft-jelly coconut milk

- 1 Burro banana

- 1/4 avocado

- 1 tablespoon date sugar or agave syrup (optional)

- 1 tablespoon chopped walnuts

Instructions:

- Begin by boiling two cups of dtlled water and adding 1 tablespoon of Dr. Seb' Nerve / Stress Relef Herbal Tea to make the anti-stress smoothie. Steep for 10 - 15 minutes, then strain and cool.

- In a high-speed blender, combine half a cup of tea with the remaining ingredients.

- Adjust sweetness if needed. Enjoy your creamy, relaxing smoothie!

17. Dr. Sebi's Orange Creamsicle Smoothie

Dr. Seb's Orange Creamsicle Smoothe helped get rid of the common cold this winter, plus it tastes exactly like an orange creamsicle! Yum!

Ingredients:

- 1 cup of coconut water
- 3 Seville oranges, peeled
- 1/2 tsp. Bromide Plus Powder
- 1/2 Burro banana
- Date sugar, to taste

Instructions:

- Add all the ingredients to your blender and blend until smooth. Serve and enjoy!

18. Green Detox Smoothie

This smoothe is high on the green stuff to help you remove any poisonous water from your body as part of the detoxification process.

Ingredients:

- 2 – 3 tbsp. key lime juice

- 1/2 burro banana

- 1/4 cup blueberries

- 1 cup Romaine lettuce

- 1/2 cup soft jelly coconut water

- 1/2 cup ginger tea

Instructions:

- Prepare tea and let cool.
- Blend all ingredients and enjoy!

19. Iron Power Smoothie

Increase the iron level in your blood with the delcou apple moothe. The "Iron Power" Smoothe will aid in the treatment of iron deficiency.

Ingredients:

- 1/2 cup cooked quinoa
- 1/2 large red apple
- 2 handfuls amaranth greens
- 1 tbsp. currants or raisins
- 1 fig
- 1 tsp. Bromide Plus Powder
- 1 cup homemade hemp seed milk
- 1 tbsp. date sugar

Instructions:

Blend everything in a high-powered blender until smooth and enjoy!

20. Dr. Sebi's Sweet Sunrise Smoothie

Ingredients:

- 1/2 burro banana
- 1 cup raspberries
- 1 cup of water
- 1 Seville orange
- 1 cup mango

Instructions:

Blend all the ingredients in a high-speed blender.

Enjoy! '

21. Dr. Sebi's "Stomach Soother" Smoothie

Cramping? Bloating? Indigestion? Pain? Soothe your stomach ache and digestive problems with Dr. Sebi's delicious Stomach Soother Smoothie!

Ingredients:

- 1 tbsp. agave syrup

- 1 burro banana

- 1/2 cup ginger tea

- 1/2 cup prepared Dr. Sebi's Stomach Relief Herbal Tea

Instructions:

Prepare tea as instructed and let cool. Blend with the remaining ingredients and enjoy!

22. Dr. Sebi's "Tropical Breeze" Smoothie

No matter how cold it is outside, this smoothie will land you in a tropical paradise!

Ingredients:

- 1/2 burro banana
- 1/2 mango
- 1 cup soft jelly coconut water
- 1/2 cup cantaloupe
- 1 handful amaranth greens
- 1/2 cup watermelon

Instructions:

- Blend all ingredients until smooth and enjoy!

23. Dr. Sebi's Energizer Smoothie

The ingredients in Dr. Seb's Energzer Smoothie will provide you with sustained energy throughout the day. Made with potent sea moss, hemp milk, nutritious grains, and fruit. Try it!

Ingredients:

- 1/2 cup cooked quinoa or amaranth
- 1 cup cubed papaya or melon
- 1 date or 1 tbsp. date sugar
- 1 cup homemade hemp milk
- 1 tsp. Bromide Plus Powder

Instructions:

Blend all the ingredients and enjoy!

24. Dr. Sebi's "Veggie-Ful" Smoothie

Ingredients:

- 1 handful watercress
- 1 pear, cored and seeded
- 1 handful Romaine lettuce
- 1/4 avocado
- 1/2 seeded cucumber, peeled
- Date sugar, to taste (optional)
- 1/2 cup spring water

Instructions:

Blend all the ingredients in a high-powered blender until smooth. Enjoy!

25. Dr. Ṣebi's "Apple Pie" Smoothie

Dr. Seb's Application Pe Smoothie tastes just like a apple pe in a cup! Try it out and let us know what you think. When the ugar cravng struck, it was perfect!

Ingredients:

- 1 cup of ginger tea
- 1/2 large apple
- 1 tsp. Bromide Plus Powder
- 2 figs
- 1 tbsp. date sugar
- Small handful walnuts

Instructions:

- Prepare the tea and allow it to cool.
- Blend all the remaining ingredients and enjoy!

26. Chamomile Delight Smoothie

Dr. Seb's Chamomile Delght Smoothe is ideal for relaxing, reducing stress, and calming your nerves before going to sleep.

Ingredients:

- 1 burro banana

- 1 tbsp. date sugar

- 1/4 cup prepared Dr. Sebi's Nerve/Stress Relief Herbal Tea

- 1/2 cup homemade walnut milk

Instructions:

- Wait for the tea to cool.
- Blend with the rest of the ingredients and enjoy!

27. Super Hydrating Smoothie

Dr. Sebi's Super Hydratng Smoothe contains natural electrolyte from the oft-jelly coconut water and ton of minerals from the watermelon and This is an excellent, refreshing option to keep you hydrated throughout the hot summer months!

Ingredients:

- 1 cup soft jelly coconut water
- 1 cup strawberries
- 1 tbsp. date sugar
- 1 cup watermelon chunks

Instructions:

Blend all ingredients and enjoy!

28. Dr. Sebi's "Brain-Boosting" Smoothie

Now that you understand the importance of caring for your brain health, it's time to try Dr. Sebi's "Brain-Boosting" Smoothie! The "Brain-Boosting" formula Smoothe contains blueberre and rapberre, which fight oxidative tre and free radical damage that causes memory malfunction. It also contains additional nutrients to provide you mental clarity and an energy boost. It's also excellent!

Ingredients:

- 1/2 cup blueberries

- 1 cup of Dr. Sebi's Nerve/Stress Relief Herbal Tea

- 1/2 burro banana

- 1/2 cup of raspberries

- 1 tablespoon of date sugar or agave syrup

Instructions:

- Begin by heating one cup of distilled water and adding 1/2 teaspoon of Dr. Sebi's Nerve / Stre Relef Herbal Tea to make your "bran-bootng" moothe. Steep for 10 - 15 minutes, then strain. Let cool.

- Once the tea is cooled, blend in a high-speed blender along with the rest of the ingredients.

- Enjoy!

29. Dr. Sebi's Heavy Metal Detox Smoothie

Do you understand the symptom of heavy metal toxicity? Heavy Metal by Dr. Sebi Detox Smoothe is properly designed to comprise x vital elements that act in synergy to clean heavy metals out of your organs where they accumulate. Begin by heating one cup of distilled water and adding 1/2 teaspoon of Dr. Sebi's Nerve / Stre Relef Herbal Tea to make your "bran-bootng" moothe. Steep for 10 - 15 minutes, then strain. Let cool.

Ingredients:

- 1 tablespoon of Dr. Sebi's Bromide Plus Powder

- 1 organic apple

- 1-2 cups blueberries

- 1 cup Seville orange juice

- 1 cup spring water

- 1 cup watercress

- 1 burro banana

Instructions:

- To make the heavy metal detox moothie, blend all ingredients in a high-powered blender until smooth.

- If a thinner consistency is desired, add up to 1 cup of water. Enjoy!

30. Dr. Sebi's "Blissful" Smoothie

Dr. Sebi's "Blissful" Smoothie is loaded with avocados. These are high in vitamin B to help keep nerve and brain cells healthy, and you a lot happier. With very clear mental and physical health benefits, this smoothie gives you all of the heartiness of the quinoa and gives you a filling and appetizing drink.

Ingredients:

- 1 oz. blueberries

- 1 pear, chopped

- 1/4 cup cooked q uinoa

- 1/4 avocado, pitted

- 1 cup of water

Instructions:

- To make your smoothie, combine all of the ingredients in a high-powered blender and enjoy!

31. Dr. Sebi's Moisturizing Hot Bath

Ingredients:

- 1 cup soft jelly coconut milk
- 2 tbsp. coconut oil
- 1 cup prepared Dr. Sebi's Nerve/Stress Relief Herbal Tea
- 15 drops avocado oil
- 1 cup of sea salt

Instructions:

- Simply add all the ingredients into a tub filled with warm water and relax!

32. Dr. Sebi's Sleepy Time Drink

Being a "night owl" carries a higher risk of mental health disorders and depression. What can you do about it? Follow these tips while sipping Dr. Seb's Sleepy Time Drnk and get ready for a good night's sleep!

Ingredients:

- 1/2 cup Dr. Sebi's Stomach Relief Herbal Tea
- 1/4 cup cooked q uinoa
- 1/4 cup cherries
- 1/2 cup Dr. Sebi's Nerve/Stress Relief Herbal Tea
- Agave syrup, to taste
- 1 burro banana
- 2 cups amaranth greens

Instructions:

- Begin by brewing the tea according to package directions to make Dr. Seb's Sleepy Tme drnk.
- Let cool.
- Blend all the ingredients in a high-speed blender and enjoy!

33. Dr. Sebi's Original "Bromide Plus" Smoothie

Ingredients:

- 1 cup fresh (approved) fruit
- 1/2 tablespoon Bromide Plus Powder
- 1 -q uart of boiling spring water
- 1/4 cup agave syrup
- 3 tablespoons walnuts

Instructions:

- To make Dr. Seb's Original Bromide Plus Smoothe, combine agave syrup, fruit, walnuts, and Bromide Plus powder in a high-powered blender.
- Slowly, add the quart of spring water, and blend for 3-4 minutes.
- Let cool, and enjoy!

33. Dr. Sebi's Pancreas-Support Smoothie

The Pancreas-Support Smoothe is packed with minerals and anti-inflammatories to provide pancreatic support from the first drink!

Ingredients:

- Juice of one key lime

- 2 cups Dr. Sebi's Stomach Relief Herbal Tea

- 1 fistful of watercress or wild arugula

- 1 tablespoon tamarind pulp

- 1 seeded cucumber

Instructions:

- Begin your Pancrea-Support Smoothie by boiling two cups dtlled water and adding 1 12 tablepoon Dr. Sebi's Stomach Relef Herbal Tea.

- Simmer for about 15 minutes. Strain and allow to cool.

- Blend the tea with the rest of the ingredients in a high-speed blender.

- Enjoy!

34. Alkaline-Mineral Smoothie

Dr. Seb's Alkalne-Mneral Smoothe is the perfect morning take: filled with alkalne mneral, fber, and uper hydrating!

Ingredients:

- 1 cup fresh spring water

- 1/2 large papaya, with seeds

- 1 tbsp. Bromide Plus Powder

- 4-5 dates

- Juice of half a key lime

- 2 burro bananas

Instructions:

To make your Alkalne-Mneral Smoothe, begin by combining all ingredients in a high-speed blender and enjoy!

35. Berry Heart-Healthy Smoothie

Now that you understand the importance of heart health, we invite you to try our Berry Heart-Healthy Smoothie. The Heart-Healthy Smoothie Recipe is ideal for a hectic morning! It's made in 5 minutes and contains nutrients that promote heart health.

Ingredients:

- 1/2 cup blueberries
- 1/2 cup raspberries
- 1 tablespoon of Bromide Plus Powder
- 1/2 cup strawberries
- 1/4 cup walnuts
- 1/2 cup blackberries

Instructions:

- Blend all ingredients on a high-speed blender and enjoy!

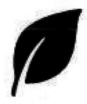

BOOK 10
Dr. Sebi's Recipes PART III

200 Delicious and Simple Recipes to Naturally Cleanse Your Liver, Lose Weight, and Lower High Blood Pressure, And Improve your health by detoxifying your body with an alkaline diet.

Soups, Stews And Sauces:
25 Recipes

1. Roasted Tomato and Bell Pepper Soup

Ingredients:

- Sesame oil
- 4 ripe Roma tomatoes
- Pure sea salt, to taste
- 3 red bell peppers
- 3 sprigs fresh thyme
- 1/4 cup homemade vegetable broth, with Dr. Sebi's approved veggies

Putting It Together:

- Scatter thyme over the vegetables.
- preheat oven to 375 degrees F.
- Drizzle generously with sesame oil and sprinkle with sea salt.
- Slice tomatoes and place onto a rimmed baking sheet with bell peppers.
- Transfer everything to a blender or food processor.
- Chop peppers into q uarters and remove centers.
- Roast in a preheated oven for 35-40 minutes.
- Add sea salt to taste. Pour into bowls and serve warm.
- Add heated broth and puree until smooth, adding more broth as necessary to reach desired consistency.

2. Chickpea Soup

Ingredients:

- 1 small onion
- 2 cups of chickpeas
- 1 bell pepper
- 1 small zucchini
- Seasoning of your choice
- Water

Instructions:

- Put everything in a pot and cook on medium heat until the vegetables are aldente.

- Once the oup and vegetable are ready, blend well with a mult - uck hand blender. It's the simplest and most enjoyable way. This recipe will create enough soup for many days.

3. Kale Soup

Ingredients:

- 1 medium onion, chopped

- 2 cups squash, diced

- 5 cups vegetable broth

- 2 teaspoons dried thyme

- 1 medium chayote, diced

- 2 teaspoons dried sage

- 3 cups kale, rinsed, stems removed and chopped very fine

- Salt and pepper to taste

Instructions:

- Chop onions and let sit for 5 minutes.

- Heat 1 tablespoon broth in a medium soup pot.

- Sauté onion in broth over medium heat for about 5 minutes stirring fr eq uently.

- Add broth, chayote, and bring to a boil.

- Once it reaches a boil, reduce the heat to a simmer and continue to cook for another 5 minutes. Cook for 15 minutes more after adding the uash.

- Cook for another 5 minutes after adding the kale and the rest of the ingredients. If you want to mer for a longer period of time for more taste and richness, add a bit more broth.

4. Alkaline Electric Soup

- 1-2 cups of Kamut Pasta/Approved Pasta
- 2 cups Butternut Squash, chopped
- 1/2 cup Quinoa (Optional)
- 1 teaspoon dill
- 1/2 lb. Garbanzo Beans (cooked)*
- 1 Small Red Onion, chopped
- 2 cups Mushrooms, chopped
- 1 Zucchini Sq uash, chopped
- 1/2 Gallon Spring Water (adjust as needed)
- 1/2 cup of chopped Red Peppers
- 1/2 cup of chopped Green Peppers
- 2 Roma Tomatoes, diced
- 1 tablespoon Sea Salt
- 1 teaspoon Basil
- 1 teaspoon Oregano
- 1 teaspoon Red Cayenne Pepper
- 1 tablespoon of Grapeseed Oil

Instructions:

- Chop up all of your vegetables.
- Pour the spring water into a large pot and turn up to medium heat.
- Stir every 15 minutes.
- Add ingredients (including seasonings) to the pot and bring to a simmer for about 1 hour.
- The leftover stew can be frozen for another time!
- Enjoy!

5. Greens Soup Recipe

Ingredients:

2 cups leafy greens

1 small zucchini

1 bell pepper

1 small onion

Water

Seasoning of your choice

Instructions:

- Put everything in a pot and cook on medium heat until the vegetables are semi-hard. Turn off the stove, let cool and blend well together.

6. Stewed Okra and Tomatoes

The recipe for Stewed Okra and Tomatoes is inexpensive, simple, and delicious! Eat it on top of uncooked or wild rice for a wonderfully nutritious alkaline-electric meal!

Ingredients:

- 1/2 cup fresh spring water

- 2 cups fresh okra

- 1 tablespoon avocado oil

- 1 cup cherry tomatoes

- 1 medium onion

- Sea salt and cayenne pepper, to taste

Instructions:

- Peel and dice the onion and cherry tomatoes.

- In a pan, heat the avacado oil and add the chopped onion. Cook until the onion becomes transparent.

- Once the onion has gone translucent, add the okra and prng water. Cook for ten minutes on low heat.

- Add the chopped cherry tomatoes and mmer for another 20 minutes, or until the okra is cooked through.

- Add sea salt and pepper, to taste.

7. Vegetable Mushroom Soup

- 1 lb oyster mushrooms, chopped
- 2 onions chopped finely
- Springwater
- 1 bunch spinach, washed and steamed
- 2 tbs olive oil
- 1/2 lb Kamut spiral pasta
- 1 small red and green bell pepper chopped
- 1 cup quinoa
- 1 clove
- 2 large chayote sq uash, peeled and chopped
- 1/2 tsp: marjoram, rosemary, oregano, thyme, red pepper, and cumin
- 2-3 bunches kale

Putting It All Together:

- Put olive oil in a hot skillet
- Simmer 45 minutes
- Add thyme, marjoram, rosemary, oregano, red pepper, cumin, clove,
- Add chayote sq uash
- Add the mushroom mixture to the soup pot and fill with spring water
- And quinoa
- Sautéed mushrooms, bell peppers, and onions slowly for 20 minutes
- Add spinach, stir, and then serve when tender
- Add kamut pasta simmer for 15 min

8. Homestyle Okra

- 1/4 tsp ground cumin
- 2 soft tomatoes
- 1/4 tsp. Sea salt
- 1/4 tsp. Sassafras
- 1/2 yellow onion chopped fine
- Alb fresh okra diced
- 4tbs olive oil
- 1/4 tsp african red pepper
- Cooked wild rice or quinoa

Instructions:

- Put everything in a pot and simmer over medium heat until the vegetables are semi-hard. Turn off the stove, allow it cool, and blend well.

9. "Zoodles" With Avocado Sauce

Ingredients

- 2 large zucchinis

- 4 tbsp key lime juice

- 2 avocados

- 1/2 cup water

- 1/2 cup walnuts

- 24 sliced cherry tomatoes

- 2 cups basil

- Sea salt, to taste.

Instructions

- Make zucchini noodles using a peeler or Spiralizer.

- Blend the remaining ingredients (excluding the cherry tomatoes) in a blender until smooth.

- Combine noodles, avocado sauce, and cherry tomatoes in a mixing bowl.

10. Xave's Delight

- 1/2 tsp. red pepper

- 2 fresh limes squeezed

- 1 oz spring water

- 3 tbs. maple syrup

- 1 tsp. sea salt

- 3 oz. sesame tahini

Putting It All Together:

- In a glass container, combine the juice of 2 limes, water, maple yrup, ea salt, and
- red pepper, and sesame tahini

11. Shake well and dress your salad!!

11. The Greatest Greens

- 3 bunches of mustard and turnips green 1/2 of each
- 1 tsp of cayenne or chili powder
- 2 cups of chopped onions
- 3 tbs sea salt
- 1/4 cup olive oil

Putting It All Together:

- Add greens, cook down for 20 min.
- Heat pan then adds onions, cook till golden brown
- Season with sea salt, and cayenne or chili powder

12. Stuffed Bell Peppers

- 1 1/2 cup of q uinoa
- 1/2 red bell peppers chopped fine
- 1 lb. oyster or brown button mushroom
- 1/2 tsp sweet basil
- 2 green bell peppers
- 3 tbs olive oil
- 1/2 tsp sea salt
- 1/4 tsp of ground cumin
- 2 slices of Kamut or spelled bread toasted, crumbled
- 1/2 tsp dill

Putting It All Together:

- Steam bell peppers until tender, then hollow out
- Season inside bell peppers with some spices and olive oil
- Place q uinoa grain in a saucepan with water covering the top
- Sauté mushrooms and red bell peppers in olive oil
- Cook low heat until water is absorbed, then set aside
- Bake in a preheated oven at 250 degrees for 10-15 minutes
- Stuff bell peppers with mixture, then sprinkle bread crumbs on top
- Mix q uinoa, mushrooms, and red bell pepper with remaining seasonings
- Serve hot and enjoy with a green leafy salad

13. Broccoli Detox Soup

A gorgeous green soup, loaded with vitamins, fiber, and minerals.

Ingredients

- 1 parsnip peeled and finely chopped
- ½ lemon juice only
- 1 onion finely diced
- Toasted mixed seeds and nuts 1 teaspoon coconut milk, to garnish
- 2 garlic cloves crushed
- 2 cups broccoli florets
- 1 cup greens kale, spinach, beet greens, or any other available
- 2 celery stalks finely diced
- 1 tsp coconut oil
- 1 carrot peeled and finely chopped
- 2 cups filtered water or low sodium vegetable broth
- ½ tsp sea salt
- 1 tbsp chia seeds

Instructions

In a soup pot, heat the coconut oil, add the onion, garlic, carrot, parsnip, celery sticks, and broccoli, and cook over low heat for five minutes, stirring fr eq uently.

Add the filtered water or vegetable broth, bring to a boil, then cover the pot with a lid and let simmer for 5-7 minutes, or until the vegetables are soft but not mushy.

Streen then tranfer to the blender, add the cha seeds and lemon, and proceen to obtan a mooth cream.

Top with toasted seeds and serve warm.

14. Beet Detox Soup

This beet oup a real powerhoue when it comes to nutrton is pnk coloured and tastes delcou.

Ingredients

- 1 tsp coconut oil

- 3 medium beetroots

- 2 carrots finely diced

- 1 tbsp chia sunflower and pumpkin seeds, 1 teaspoon coconut milk, to garnish

- 2 cups vegetable broth warm

- 1 onion finely diced

- ¼ tsp sea salt

- 2 garlic cloves crushed

- 1 small leek finely diced

Instructions

- Place the unpeeled beetroots in a pot, cover with water, bring to boil then simmer for 30 minutes until tender.

- Drain from water and set aside to cool.

- Heat the coconut oil in a skillet, then add the onion, garlic, leek, and carrot and cook for 5-7 minutes over low heat. Remove yourself from the heat and transfer to a plate.

- Peel the beetroots, cut into cubes, and add to the blender with the cooked veggies and warm vegetable broth.

- The process to obtain a smooth cream.
- Season with salt and serve garnished with mixed seeds.

15. Sweet Potato Detox Soup

Ingredients

- ½ cup cooked red lentils

- 1 tsp turmeric powder

- 1 sweet potato peeled and cut into cubes

- 3 garlic cloves crushed

- 3 carrots peeled and roughly chopped

- 1 onion peeled and cut into quarters

- 1 parsnip peeled and roughly chopped

- ¼ tsp sea salt

- Pinch of chili powder

- 1 tsp cumin powder

- 1/2 inch piece of ginger peeled and grated

- Fresh parsley 1 teaspoon coconut milk, to garnish

- 1 tsp coconut oil

- 2 cups low sodium vegetable broth warm

Instructions

- Heat the oven at 165°C/329°F.

- Line a bakng heet wth bakng paper, add the sweet potato, carrot, parnp, onon, and garlc, season wth alt, chl, turmerc, and cumn, add the coconut oil, and

- Roast for 20 minutes then transfers into the blender.

- Add the warm vegetable broth, grated ginger, and cooked red lentils to the blender and blend until smooth.

- Serve warm, garnished with fresh parsley.

- Packed with vitamin A and fibre, the orange out the best chooe for a detox dinner.

16. Spice And Seed Mix For Detox Soups

Use this spices mix whenever you want toa dd a new flavor to any of your detox soups.

Ingredients

- 1 cup hazelnuts lightly toasted, crushed
- 1/2 tsp cinnamon ground
- 2 tsp nigella seeds
- 1/4 tsp coriander seeds crushed
- 2 tsp sesame seeds
- 1 tsp turmeric
- 1/2 cup pumpkin seeds
- 1/4 tsp garlic powder
- 1/2 tsp cayenne pepper
- 1/4 tsp ginger powder

Instructions

- Add all the ingredients into a jar with lid, mix to combine.
- Add 2 tsp of the mix on top of a soup serving.

17. Chicken Chili Soup

Ingredient

- ½ teaspoon ground cumin
- 1 tablespoon dried parsley
- ½ cup frozen corn kernels
- 2 teaspoons chili powder
- 2 medium (blank)s red bell peppers, diced
- 4 (15 ounce) cans kidney beans with l iq uid
- 2 (14.5 ounces) cans diced tomatoes
- 1 onion, diced
- 2 cups of water
- ½ teaspoon ground cayenne pepper
- 2 medium (blank)s green bell peppers, diced
- 1 teaspoon garlic powder
- 1 (15 ounces) can tomato sauce
- 1 ¾ pound diced chicken breast meat

Instructions

Coat a big pot with cooking spray and set it over medium-high heat. Cook and stir chicken, bell pepper, and one until chicken brown and pepper are just tender. Stir in corn, beans, tomatoes, tomato sauce, and water. Seaon with chl powder, parley, garlc powder, cayenne, and cumn. Reduce heat, cover, and simmer for 30 minutes.

18. Healthier Slow Cooker Chicken And Dumplings

Ingredients

- 4 chicken breast halves, bone and kn removed (blank)s knle, boneless
- 10 ounces refrigerated reduced-fat biscuit dough, torn into pieces
- 1 cup frozen peas
- 3 carrot, (7-1/2")s carrots, sliced
- 1 onion, finely diced
- 2 tablespoons butter
- 2 cups natural cream of chicken soup

Instruction

- Place chicken, butter, cream of chicken soup, and onion in a slow cooker. Cover and cook on High for 5 to 6 hours. Stir in carrots after 5 hours of cooking.
- 30 minutes before serving, the spot was torn biscuit dough in a slow cooker. Cook for about 25 minutes, or until the centre is no longer raw. Lft biscuit edges and stir in pea. Allow to warm for about 10 minutes before serving.

19. Chicken Tortilla Soup

Ingredients

- ½ cup chopped fresh cilantro
- 2 breast half, bone and skin removed (blank)s skinless, boneless chicken breast halves, cut into bite-size pieces
- 1 (15 ounces) can whole kernel corn, drained
- ½ teaspoon ground cumin
- ½ teaspoon chili powder
- ½ teaspoon dried oregano
- 1 (15 ounces) can black beans, rinsed and drained
- 3 cups chicken broth
- 6 (6 inches) corn tortillas, cut into 1/2 inch strips
- ½ cup of salsa
- 2 ½ teaspoons vegetable oil

Instruction

- In a big saucepan, heat 2 teaspoons of oil over medium heat. Add half of the tortilla strips and toss often until crisp. Dran on a paper towel Repeat with the remaining 1/2 teaspoon of ol and remaining tortlla trp and set aside.

- Pour in the broth, cumin, chilli powder, and oregano. Raise the heat to high and bring to a boil. Add the bean, corn, cheddar, and ala. Reduce heat to low, stir, and simmer for about 2 minutes, or until chicken is cooked through and no longer pink on the outside.

- Add the cinnamon and half of the saved tortlla strp. Ladle into ndvdual bowls and garnh each bowl wth ome of the remanng trp.

20. Spicy Slow Cooker Black Bean Soup

Ingredients

- ¾ teaspoon ground black pepper

- 1 teaspoon ground cumin

- 4 teaspoons diced jalapeno peppers

- ½ teaspoon hot pepper sauce

- ½ teaspoon garlic powder

- 1 tablespoon chili powder

- 1 teaspoon cayenne pepper

- 6 cups chicken broth

- 1 pound dry black beans, soaked overnight

Instruction

- Drain black beans, and rinse.

- In a slow cooker, combine bean, jalapeno, and chicken broth. Season with garlc powder, chl powder, cumin, cayenne pepper, pepper, and hot pepper auce.

- Cook on High for 4 hours. Reduce the heat to low and continue cooking for 2 hours, or until you're ready to eat.

21. Chunky Vegetarian Vegetable Soup (Fast And Easy)

Ingredient

- 2 eaches baking potatoes, cut into bite-size pieces
- 4 cups vegetable broth
- 1 cup frozen shelled edamame (green soybeans)
- 1 cup frozen sliced okra
- ½ onion, chopped
- 2 leaves kale, roughly chopped
- 4 medium (blank)s carrots, peeled and cut into 1/4-inch rounds
- 2 tablespoons olive oil
- 1 cup of frozen corn
- 1 teaspoon ground black pepper
- 2 cloves garlic, minced
- 1 (15 ounces) can tomato sauce
- salt to taste
- 3 stalks celery, chopped

Instruction

- Heat olive oil in a large pot over medium heat. Cook and stir onion and celery in hot oil for 5 minutes, or until softened and translucent.
- Stir garlic into the onion mixture; cook and stir until fragrant, 2 to 3 minutes more.
- Pour vegetable broth and tomato sauce into the pot. Simmer for about 10 minutes.
- Stir the carrot and potato through the broth. Simmer for 10 to 15 minutes more, or until the carrots are soft..

Drop corn, edamame, okra, and kale into the soup. Continue to simmer until okra is tender, 5 to 10 minutes more. Season with salt and pepper.

22. Chinese Chicken Vegetable Soup

Ingredients

- 1 teaspoon vegetable oil
- □½ teaspoon Asian (toasted) sesame oil
- ½ red bell pepper, chopped
- 1 stalk celery, thinly sliced
- 1 (7 ounces) can baby corn ears
- 1 cup shredded napa cabbage
- 1 teaspoon minced fresh ginger root
- 1 cup sliced fresh mushrooms
- 1 cup snow peas
- 1 chicken bouillon cube
- 1 (8 ounces) can sliced water chestnuts, rinsed and drained
- 1 (10 ounces) bag shredded carrots
- 1 cup broccoli florets
- 1 clove garlic, minced
- 1 skinless, boneless chicken breast half - cut into bite-size pieces
- 5 eaches green onions, chopped
- 8 cups of water
- 1 small zucchini, thinly sliced
- 1 pound boneless chicken thighs - cut into bite-size pieces
- 2 teaspoons soy sauce

Instruction

- Heat the vegetable oil in a large Dutch oven or a large pot over medium-high heat, and cook and stir the chicken until it is no longer pink, about 3 minutes. When the chicken is cooked, add the water, chicken bouillon cube, ginger, soy sauce, and eame oil. Bring to a boil, then decrease heat to a simmer.

- Stir in the baby corn, water chestnut, carrot, broccoli floret, napa cabbage, red bell pepper, green onion, celery, zucchini, and new peas, and simmer for 1 to 2 minutes, or until the carrot softens and the broccoli and new peas turn bright green. Mix in the mushrooms and cook for another 5 minutes.

23. Vegan Tomato Soup

Ingredients

- ¾ cup vegetable broth
- 2 sprigs fresh basil, divided
- 4 cloves garlic, minced
- 2 eaches bay leaves
- 3 ½ cups cherry tomatoes, halved
- 2 tablespoons extra-virgin olive oil
- 4 medium whole (2-3/5" dia) (blank)s tomatoes, chopped
- 1 onion, chopped

Instruction

- In a saucepan, heat olive oil over low heat and cook one at a time until soft and transformant. Cook until the garlc is fragrant, about 1 minute. Increase the heat to medium, add all of the tomatoes, and simmer until they begin to break down, about 5 minutes. Occasionally, str. Add vegetable broth, bay leaves, and 1 sprig bal. Bring to a boil, then reduce heat and simmer for 30 minutes, or until the tomatoes have broken down and the soup has begun to thicken.

- Remove soup from heat and cool slightly. Remove bay leaves and basil.

- Puree tomato soup with an immersion blender until smooth. Reheat soup before serving and garnish with basil leaves.

24. Slow Cooker Mediterranean Stew

Ingredients

- 1 clove garlic, chopped
- ¼ teaspoon paprika
- 1 carrot, sliced thin
- 2 cups cubed zucchini
- ¼ teaspoon crushed red pepper
- 1 cup chopped onion
- 1 ripe tomato, chopped
- ¼ teaspoon ground cinnamon
- ½ cup vegetable broth
- ⅓ cup raisins
- ½ teaspoon ground turmeric
- ½ teaspoon ground cumin
- 1 butternut squash - peeled, seeded, and cubed
- 1 (8 ounces) can tomato sauce
- 1 (10 ounces) package frozen okra, thawed
- 2 cups cubed eggplant, with peel

Instruction

- Combine butternut uah, eggplant, zucchini, okra, tomato sauce, onon, tomato, carrot, broth, ran, and garlic in a slow cooker. Season with cumin, turmeric, red pepper flakes, cinnamon, and paprika.
- Cover, and cook on Low for 8 to 10 hours, or until vegetables are tender.

25. Smooth Broccoli Vitamin Soup

Ingredients

⅛ teaspoon ground thyme

⅛ teaspoon ground black pepper

⅛ teaspoon of sea salt

1 head broccoli, cut into florets

1 cup milk

1 cup chicken broth

½ small onion, diced

2 medium (2-1/4" to 3" dia, raw)s potatoes, diced

⅛ teaspoon ground ginger

1 ½ teaspoon olive oil

Instruction

- Heat olive oil in a skillet over medium heat; saute onion until translucent, 5 to 10 minutes.

- Spread potatoes and broccoli onto a microwave-safe plate. Cook in the microwave until tender, 4 to 5 minutes.

- Place the onion, potato, broccoli, milk, chicken broth, pepper, salt, ginger, and thyme in the Vitamix or blender. Begin on variable 1, gradually progress to variable 10, and finish on high for 4 to 5 minutes. Serve hot.

Sea Moss Recipes And Mushroom Recipes All Joined; 20 Recipes

Dr. Sebi Approved Sea Moss Recipes Of All Time

You may recall Dr. Sebi giving credit to something called 'ea mo' for assisting him to father 17 children. The sea is so densely filled with nutrients that benefit male health in particular, that some brothers have thrown away their Vagra! Whether you have a problem in that area or not, ea mo should be on everyone's menu - women and men alike. That's because sea moss is high in vitamins, minerals, and nutrients such as:

- Dietary fiber
- Vitamin K
- Calcium
- Copper
- Riboflavin
- Folate
- Iron
- Magnesium
- Phosphorus
- Zinc
- Iodine
- Sulfur
- Manganese.

And because it is an algae, it is suitable for all plant-based diets, including the Melanin Diet. The issue with ea mo is that it is not very appetising on its own. The taste and texture are a big turn-off. The good news is that there are some delicious recipes out there that will have you desiring sea moss every day of the week. Before you check out the recipe, you should have some eental on hand and ready to begin. Here are the tools and resources I recommend.

How To Prepare Sea Moss

Before you begin with the ea moss recipes below, you must first transform the raw mo from its solid state to a gel or paste. Here is how to prepare your sea mo according to the instructions in our original post here.

Step 1: Remove your sea moss from the bag and wash it thoroughly.

Step 2: Put it into a large bowl filled with cool water. It doesn't look like a lot but this stuff expands so make sure to use a large bowl filled with water.

Step 3: Cover and leave overnight to rehydrate. Once the sea moss has absorbed the water in the bowl, it will look something like this...

Step 4: Put your sea moss into a blender along with 1 cup of activated water for every ounce of sea moss

Step 5: You now have a sea moss jelly that you can put in a mason jar and store in the refrigerator for up to 3 weeks or use immediately.

1. Sea Moss Recipe – Sweet Vegan Sea Moss Smoothie Recipe

Here is a great vegan sea moss recipe from Charla that is so good you can drink it all day!

Ingredients

- 1 tsp of Vanilla

- 6 cups warm water (to soak the moss)

- 1/8 tsp Nutmeg

- Coconut condensed milk (optional to taste)

- 1 cup nut milk (can use coconut milk)

- 1/4 cup of coconut nectar

- 2 tbsp of linseed

- 1/8 tsp Cinnamon

- 100g of sea moss

Instructions

- Place the sea moss in a colander.

- Use your hands to thoroughly wash away any debris and excess salt from your moss. Do this many times until the ea moss looks and feels gritty.

- Place the sea moss and flaxeed in a large basin with 6 cups of warm water and leave to soak overnight. The moss will grow in size, and the water level will rise somewhat.

- Use a colander to pour and drain off the excess water that was used to soak the sea moss

- Put the sea moss in a blender bowl and purée it into a paste. The sea should be gelatnou n texture. Don't worry, it's not very thick to begin with; if you store it in a big jar in the refrigerator, it will turn thick over time.

- Scoop out the paste and transfer into a jar/bowl and refrigerate.

- In a high-powered blender, combine 4 tablespoons of the ea moss paste with the almond milk, vanilla, spices, and sweetener of your choice.

- Serve

2. Sea Moss Recipe – Chef Sian's Sea Moss Shake Recipe

This recipe comes from Chef Sian.

Ingredients

- 4 oz Sea Moss
- 1 tsp vanilla
- 2 TB linseed
- ¼ tsp grated ginger
- 3 q ts water
- ¼ tsp cinnamon
- ¼ C. isinglass

Instructions

- In a large pot, combine Irih mo, isinglass, Ineed, and water. After the Irh moss has been boiled, use a tranner to transfer the liquid to a bowl. Allow the transported l ud to cool. The liquid will congeal. In a blender, combine 14 of the gel with the remaining ingredients and mx for 3 to 4 minutes. Chill for 2 to 4 hours before serving. If the drink is too thick for your liking, add 12 cup water to the blender and then beverage.

- Freeze unused Irish moss in a container or freezer bag for up to 3 months and use as needed

3. Sea Moss Recipe – Jamaican Country Style Irish Moss Drink Recipe

Ingredients

- ☐3 pieces of gum arabic

- 1 teaspoon ground nutmeg

- 3/4 cup date sugar

- 1/4 cup ground linseed

- 6 strands isinglass

- 2 ounces Irish moss

- 2 cups Coconut Milk

- 2 teaspoons Vanilla Flavoring

- 3 large ice cubes, or about 1/4 cup very cold water

Instructions

- Combine the coconut milk, moss, and ice cubes in a blender and blend well.

- Heat 2 cups water in a saucepan over medium heat with the milk, 1/3 cup of the Irh mo combination, the lneed, ngla, and gum arabc.

- Bring to a boil and simmer for 30 minutes, or until all of the ingredients have been dissolved and integrated and the sauce has thickened.

- On low heat and add the date sugar, vanilla, and nutmeg and continue cooking, stirring occasionally for another 10 minutes.

- Take the pan off the heat. If you want it cold, put it in the refrigerator for 3 hours. It will generally thicken and cool.

4. Sea Moss Recipe – Fruit Smoothie Sea Moss Recipes

Ingredients

- 1 banana
- 1/4 cup coconut water
- 2 tbsp Hemp seeds)
- 1 thumb ginger
- 1 peeled orange
- 1/2 cup African mango
- 1/2 cup cherries
- 2 pitted dates
- 1 apple
- 1/2 thumb turmeric
- 1/4 cup sea moss gel
- 1 cup strawberries
- 1/2 cup pineapple

Instructions

Freeze the mango, banana, pineapple, and strawberries first.

Place all ingredients into blender and mix until smooth.

Enjoy!!!

5. Sea Moss Recipe – L iq uid Viagra

Ingredients

- 3 tbsp. vanilla extract
- Black Strap Molasses
- 5 oz. linseed
- 3 oz. gum arabic
- 5 oz. isinglass
- 1 cup of raw organic natural honey
- 2 tablespoons of powdered nutmeg
- 5 qt. water
- ¾ lb Irish Moss

Instructions

- Pour the liquid into a strainer into another container. Throw away the boiled Irish Moss.
- Add Irish Moss, gum arabic, isinglass, and linseed.
- Add the rest of the ingredients to the liquid and mix well. Boil for an additional 10 minutes.
- Place 5 qt. water in a pot and bring to a boil
- Cook for ¾ hour until all the ingredients, except the Irish Moss, has dissolved.
- Let the mixture cool and then place in the refrigerator for 5 hours before severing.

6. Sea Moss Panna Cotta!

Ingredients:

- ¼ cup + 1 tablespoon coconut oil
- ¼ cup agave syrup
- 1 tablespoon of Bromide Plus Powder
- ½ heaping cup soft-jelly young coconut meat
- 2 cups + 2 tablespoons soft-jelly coconut water
- Pinch unrefined sea salt
- 2/3 cup soaked walnuts

Instructions:

- Begin preparing your ea mo panna cotta by blendng the soaked walnut and oft-jelly coconut water (ideally in a high-peed blender). Blend at medium-high speed until smooth. Pour through a nut milk bag or a strainer lined with a double layer of cheesecloth. Squeeze to remove as much liquid as possible.

- Place the walnut milk you just made, Bromide Plu Powder, oft-jelly coconut meat, and agave syrup in a high-speed blender.

- Blend at medium speed first, then raise to high speed until completely smooth. This will take 1 to 2 minutes. Ensure that the mixture is entirely smooth.

- Greate the insides of 6 ramekins, moulds, or epreo cups with coconut oil (no need to greate if serving in the ramekins/cups). Pour mxture n to fill to the desired height. Chill your ea mo panna cotta in the refrigerator for at least 2 hours, or until set and firm.

- Add strawberries and agave syrup to taste before serving. Enjoy!

7. One-Pot Zucchini Mushroom Pasta

Now that you know everything there is to know about the incredible health advantages of mushroom and why you should include it in your diet, it is time to try Dr. Seb's One-Pot Zucchn Muhroom Pata! This One-Pot Zucchini Muhroom Pata recipe will save you time and money, and it's delicious.

Ingredients:

- Sea salt and cayenne pepper, to taste

- 2 sprigs thyme

- 2 zucchini, thinly sliced and quartered

- 1 pound cremini mushrooms, thinly sliced

- 1 pound approved-grain spaghetti (like spelled or Kamut)
- 1/4 cup homemade walnut milk

Instructions:

- Combine paghett, mushrooms, zucchini, and thyme in a large tockpot or Dutch oven over medium-high heat; season with sea salt and cayenne pepper to taste.

- Bring to a boil; decrease heat and simmer, uncovered, for 8-10 minutes, or until pasta is cooked through and liquid has been reduced.

- Stir in homemade walnut milk.
- Serve immediately and enjoy it.

8. Dr. Sebi's Mushroom Risotto

This is the best mushroom risotto! It's rich, creamy, and brimming with flavour! Try Dr. Sebi's Muhroom Rotto for a delectable and elegant evening.

Ingredients:

- 2 cups wild rice
- 4 mushrooms
- 1 tbsp. grapeseed oil
- Cayenne pepper, to taste
- 1/2 onion
- Sea salt, to taste
- 4 cups homemade vegetable broth (made from approved vegetables)

Instructions:

- Cook mushrooms and one tablespoon grapeseed oil in a large saucepan over medium heat. Cook for 5 to 7 minutes, or until the mushrooms are lightly browned and the liquid has evaporated, stirring occasionally.
- Stir in rice and cook an additional minute.
- Add the veggie broth, sea salt, and pepper to taste. Cover and cook for 2 hours and 45 minutes on low heat or 1 hour 15 minutes on high heat, or until rice is tender.

9. Plant-Based Mushroom Gravy!

Ingredients:

- 2 tablespoons of finely chopped walnuts
- 1/2 cup homemade (approved) vegetable broth
- 1 cup thinly sliced mushrooms (any type, except shiitake)
- 1/2 teaspoon fresh thyme
- 1 1/2 tablespoons amaranth or spelled flour
- 1 cup homemade walnut milk
- 1/4 of an onion, diced
- 2 tablespoons grapeseed oil
- 1 pinch each sea salt and cayenne pepper

Instructions:

- In a cast-iron skillet or big saucepan, heat the grapeseed oil over medium heat. Then add the on and muhroom and season with a pinch of ea alt and cayenne pepper. Cook, stirring occasionally, for 3-4 minutes, or until the onions are soft.
- Add amaranth or spelled flour and whisk to coat. Cook for 1 minute.
- Then gradually include homemade vegetable broth and walnut milk, starting with 1/2 cup and progressively increasing. Seaon once more with a pinch of each ea salt and cayenne pepper. Over low heat, cook until thickened, stirring often. Spices should be tasted and adjusted as needed.
- Add the walnuts and whisk to combine. Continue to cook on low until ready to serve, adding more walnut milk as required if it gets too thick.
- Serve over plant-based biscuits or bread made with flour from approved grains.

10. T aq uitos

- 2 tbs oregano

- 2 tsp. onion powder

- 2 tsp. ground thyme

- 3 tbs sea salt

- 2 tbs tomato sauce

- 2 cups of chopped onion

- 4 cups of chopped mushrooms

- 2 tsp chili powder

Putting It All Together:

- Add mushroom sauté for 5 minutes

- Wrap in corn shells tightly

- Add 1/4 cup of olive oil to the pan

- Then add seasonings

- Add onion sauté until golden brown

- Then fry until crispy

11. Mushroom Salad

- 1/4 bunch red leaf lettuce, torn
- 1/4 cup fresh lime juice
- 1/4 bunch romaine lettuce, torn
- 1/2 lb. fresh mushrooms
- 1/2 red bell pepper, chopped
- 1/2 cup olive oil
- 1 sm. red onion, diced
- 1/4 bunch fresh spinach, torn
- 1/2 tsp. dill
- 1/2 tsp. basil
- 1/2 tsp. sea salt

Putting It All Together:

- Thoroughly wash greens, dry and shred
- Place greens with mushrooms and mix thoroughly
- Marinade 1/2 hour in the refrigerator
- Thoroughly wash mushrooms, dry, slice
- Add onion, bell pepper, olive oil, lime juice, dill, sea salt, and basil
- Enjoy!

12. Spaghetti Recipe

- Follow Instructions: on the Vita Spelt Pasta box on how to cook the

- pasta.

- After the pasta is cooked, strain it.

- In a separate pan add 1/2 cup of olive oil

- Heat sauce on medium-high for 10 minutes

- add 4 tbs of sea salt

- 1 1/2 tbs of onion powder

- 2 tbs of cayenne/chili powder

- 3 tbs of maple syrup

- 2 cups of tomato sauce

- Stir pasta into the sauce

- Let sit for 5 minutes.

Instructions:

Serve and Enjoy!

13. Lasagna

- 2 tbs olive oil
- 2 lb., mushrooms
- 1 red bell pepper, chopped
- Bay leaf, crumbled
- Spelled lasagna pasta
- 1 yellow onion chopped
- Oregano, to taste
- Almond cheddar cheese
- 8 fresh tomatoes
- Sea salt, to taste

Putting It All Together:

Tomato Sauce

- Heat a skillet and add olive oil
- Blend tomato in a blender -fresh tomato sauce
- Season to taste sauté for 2 minutes and add 1/2 of saved sauce
- Boil tomatoes for 10 minutes
- Place in ice water for five minutes, drain and remove the skin from tomatoes
- remaining half to be used when layering.
- Add tomato sauce in a skillet with sautéed seasonings
- Simmer for 30-45 minutes
- Set aside half of the sauce to be used to make the mushroom sauce,
- Place onion, bell peppers, oregano, sea salt, and bay leaf in skillet
- Mushroom sauce
- Place mushrooms in water, soak for 1 minute, strain and slice
- and sauté
- (see above), set aside for layering.

Pasta

- Place a layer of pasta on top then a layer of mushroom sauce

- ☐Prepare pasta according to instructions

- Layer a deep baking dish with tomato sauce

- Repeat steps until the dish are almost full

- Then add a layer of almond cheddar

- Once pasta is done, place under cold water for easy handling

- Bake in a 350-degree oven for 20 minutes until almond cheddar is melted

- Place 2 cups of sauce on top of the remainder of almond cheddar

14. Hot Veggie Wrap

- 3 cups diced tomatoes

- 1 cup of diced bell peppers

- 2 cups onion

- 1/2 cup of mushrooms chopped

Putting It All Together:

- Stir fry all vegetables for 5 minutes

- Warm spelled tortilla

- Put together

- Enjoy!

15. Wild Rice

- Wild rice
- 1/8 tsp. African red pepper
- 1 medium yellow onion chopped fine
- 2 tsp. oregano
- 1 cup mushrooms, chopped medium, fine (oyster or brown button)
- 1/8 cup olive oil
- 1 tsp. thyme
- 1 small red pepper
- 1 tsp. sea salt
- Springwater

Putting It All Together:

- Sauté vegetables and mushrooms 2-3 minutes
- Fold in Cooked rice and simmer for 20 minutes
- pour olive oil in a hot skillet
- Soak rice in spring water overnight for best results
- Add thyme, oregano, sea salt, and African red pepper
- Cook rice according to package instructions and set aside

Tip: If you forget to soak rice overnight:

- Parboil rice for 20 minutes set aside loosely covered until rice opens
- (approx. 2-3 hours)
- Rinse and cook until tender
- Or:
- Boil rice, adding additional water, and stirring as needed until tender.

16. Spaghetti Recipe

- Follow directions on the Vita Spelt Pasta box on how to cook the pasta.

- After the pasta is cooked, strain it.

- In a separate pan add 1/2 cup of olive oil

- 2 cups of tomato sauce

- add 4 tbs of sea salt

- 1 1/2 tbs of onion powder

- 2 tbs of cayenne/chili powder

- 3 tbs of maple syrup

- Heat sauce on medium-high for 10 minutes

- Stir pasta into the sauce

- Let sit for 5 minutes.

Instructions

Serve and Enjoy!

17. Sea Moss Drink (Irish Moss Drink)

Ingredients

- To make the sea moss gel
- 6 cups warm water to soak the moss
- 100 g of Jamaican Irish moss/sea moss
- 2 tbsp of linseed flaxseed

To Make The Drink

- Coconut condensed milk optional to taste
- 1 cup Almond milk can use coconut milk
- 1/4 cup of Sweetener - coconut nectar agave nectar, maple syrup
- 1/8 tsp Cinnamon
- 1/8 tsp Nutmeg
- 1 tsp of Vanilla

Instructions

- Place the sea moss in a colander.
- Using your hands, carefully wah any debr and exce ea alt from your mo. Do this several times until the sea moss looks and feels gritty.
- Place the sea mo and flaxeed in a large bowl with 6 cups of warm water and let to soak overnight. The moss will grow in size, and the water level will rise somewhat.
- Use a colander to pour and drain off the excess water that was used to soak the sea moss
- Pour the ea mo into a blender bowl and purée on a plate. The ea mo should have a gelatnou texture. Don't worry, it's not very thick to begin with, but if you store it in a big jar in the refrigerator, it will thicken with time.
- Scoop out the paste and transfer into a jar/bowl and refrigerate.
- In a high-speed blender, combine 4 tablespoons of the ea mo paste with the almond milk, vanilla, spices, and sweetener of your choice.
- Blend into a smooth consistency - add any extra i.e rum, stout, oats, etc.. now if r eq uired

- Serve accordingly.

Notes

- Some individuals keep their mogel in the refrigerator for up to four weeks. I recommend keeping it for 3-4 days for maximum potency.

- For longevity freeze the gel into small ice cubes.

- DO NOT USE powdered or flaked ea mo, the form of mo is refned and has lost its nutritious value.

- You can also use this recipe to make the sea moss gel only for additional purposes

- To make a single glass of the drink, use 1/3 cup of monadad soaked in 2-3 cups of water and follow the rest of the directions.

- Make sure the sea moss you are using is "Wildcrafted" or "Wild Harvested".

- It is normal for the moss gel to thicken up as it is refrigerated.

- If the actual drink is too thick, add a splash of almond milk

18. Jazzed Up Apple Smoothie

Ingredients

- 1 dash ground cinnamon
- 1 tbsp. sea moss gel
- 1 dash ground cloves
- 1 banana frozen
- 1 tbsp. fresh ginger
- 2 c. fresh-pressed apple juice
- 2 c. ice cubes

Instructions

- Place all ingredients in your blender and pulse until smooth. Serve and enjoy!

19. Raw Cacao Smoothie

Ingredients

- 1 dash cinnamon
- 1 dash nutmeg
- 1 banana frozen
- 4-6 Medjool dates pitted
- 2-4 tbsp. raw cacao powder
- 4 c. almond milk
- 1 pinch Himalayan Pink Crystal salt
- 1 tbsp. coconut butter/oil
- ½ oz. prepared Irish Moss
- ½ vanilla bean scraped or sub with 1 tbsp. vanilla extract

Instructions

- Add all of the ingredients to your blender and mix until creamy! You may change the consistency of your smoothie by adjusting the amount of mo. Drink and have fun!

20. Prepared Sea Moss

Ingredients

- 1½-2 c. Springwater
- 1 c. Sea Moss

Instructions

- Begin by rnng a handful of mo. Expect it for ea debr, and, and other defect. When it is clean and ready, immerse it in enough water to cover it for 4-24 hours at room temperature. Every 4-6 hours, rinse the moss and change the water. The ea moss should become transparent, velvety, and double in size. When this occurs, drain and rinse one more.

- Then, combine the prepared sea moss with the spring water in a blender and blend until smooth and creamy. Place the mixture in an airtight container and refrigerate for at least an hour, or until it thickens.

BOOK 11
Dr. Sebi's Recipes PART IV

200 Delicious and Simple Recipes to Naturally Cleanse Your Liver, Lose Weight, and Lower High Blood Pressure, And Improve your health by detoxifying your body with an alkaline diet.

Grains And Main Dishes:
30 Recipes

1. Oatmeal-Rhubarb Porridge

Ingredients

- 1 cup old-fashioned rolled oats

- ½ teaspoon ground cinnamon

- 1 ½ cups 1 1/2 cups nonfat milk or nondairy milk, such as soymilk or almond milk

- 1 cup 1/2-inch pieces rhubarb, fresh or frozen

- ½ cup of orange juice

- 1 pinch Pinch of salt

- 2 tablespoons chopped pecans or other nuts, toasted (see Tip) if desired

- 3 tablespoons 2-3 tablespoons brown sugar, pure maple syrup or agave syrup

Instructions

- Blend milk, juice, oatmeal, rhubarb, cinnamon, and salt in a medium aucepan. Bring to a boil on medium-high heat. Reduce heat, cover, and cook at a very gentle bubble, stirring frequently, until the oatmeal and rhubarb are tender, about 5 minutes. Remove from the heat and let aside for 5 minutes, covered. To taste, add sweetener. Finish with nuts.

Tip: To toast chopped nuts, place in a small dry kettle and cook over medium-low heat, stirring constantly, for 2 to 4 minutes, or until crisp and lightly browned. People with celiac disease or gluten sensitivity should consume "gluten-free" oats, as oats are frequently mixed with wheat and barley.

2. Buddha Bowl

Ingredients

- 1 teaspoon extra-virgin olive oil

- 1 cup small cauliflower florets

- 1 tablespoon lemon juice

- 2 tablespoons tahini

- 3 tablespoons hot tap water

- ¼ teaspoon salt, divided

- ½ teaspoon ground cumin

- 1 teaspoon za'atar

- 1 clove garlic, minced

- ½ cup canned chickpeas, rinsed

- ½ cup cooked q uinoa

- 1 ½ cups baby kale

Instructions

- Preheat oven to 425 degrees F.

- In a medium bowl, combine the cauliflower, oil, cumin, and 1/8 teaspoon salt. Transfer to a small baking dish and bake for 12 to 15 minutes, or until the cauliflower is tender.

- Meanwhile, in a separate bowl, whisk together the water, tahini, lemon juice, garlc, za'atar, and the remaining 1/8 teaspoon tea.

- Fill a large serving dish halfway with kale. Top with cauliflower, quinoa, and chickpeas; drizzle with 2 tablespoons of the dressing (save the rest for another use).

3. Oatmeal

Ingredients

- ⅓ cup dried cranberries
- ⅓ cup dried apricots, chopped
- 8 cups of water
- 2 cups steel-cut oats, (see Ingredient note)
- ¼ teaspoon salt, or to taste

Instructions

- In a 5- or 6-quart slow cooker, combine water, oats, dried cranberries, dried apricots, and salt. Reduce the heat to low. Cook for 7 to 8 hours, or until the oatmeal is tender and the batter is creamy.

- Stovetop Variation

- Reduce the following recipe to accommodate the size of typical double boilers: In a double boiler, combine 4 cups water, 1 cup steel-cut oatmeal, 3 teaspoons dried cranberries, 3 tablespoons dried apricot, and 1/8 teaspoon salt. Cook for about 1 1/2 hours over boiling water, checking the water level in the bottom of the double boiler from time to time.

4. Warm Quinoa Salad With Edamame & Tarragon

Ingredients

- 2 tablespoons extra-virgin olive oil
- 2 tablespoons lemon juice
- 2 cups frozen shelled edamame, thawed (10 ounces)
- 2 tablespoons chopped fresh tarragon or 2 teaspoons dried
- 2 cups vegetable broth
- 1 cup quinoa, (see Note)
- 1 tablespoon freshly grated lemon zest
- ¼ cup 1/4 cup chopped walnuts, preferably toasted (see Cooking Tip)
- ½ cup 1/2 cup drained and diced jarred roasted red peppers, (3 ounces)
- ½ teaspoon salt

Instructions

- Toast q uinoa in a dry skillet over medium heat, stirring often, until it becomes aromatic and begins to crackle about 5 minutes. Transfer to a fine sieve and rinse thoroughly.

- In a medium saucepan over high heat, bring the broth to a boil. Return to a boil after adding the unoa. Cover, reduce heat to a simmer, and cook for 8 minutes. Remove the old and, without disturbing the unoa, add edamame. Cook until the edamame and quinoa are soft, about 7 to 8 minutes longer. If necessary, dran any remaining water.

- In a large bowl, combine lemon zest and juice, oil, tartargon, and salt. Add the pepper and quinoa mixture. to put together Divide across 4 plates and top with walnuts.

5. Lemon-Parm Popcorn

Ingredients

- 1 tablespoon freshly grated Parmesan cheese
- 3 cups air-popped popcorn
- 1 pinch Pinch of salt
- ½ teaspoon lemon pepper
- 2 teaspoons extra-virgin olive oil

Instructions

- In a small bowl, combine the ol, lemon pepper, and salt. Drizzle over popcorn and to coat. Serve immediately after sprinkling with Parmesan.

6. Bacony Barley Salad With Marinated Shrimp

Ingredients

- 3 piece (blank)s 3 strips bacon, chopped
- ⅔ cup quick-cooking barley
- ½ teaspoon salt
- 1 ⅓ cups water
- 1 pound peeled cooked shrimp, (21-25 per pound; thawed if frozen), tails removed, coarsely chopped
- 2 cups cherry tomatoes, halved
- ⅓ cup lime juice
- 2 tablespoons extra-virgin olive oil
- ½ cup chopped fresh cilantro
- 1 avocado, peeled and diced
- 1 Freshly ground pepper, to taste
- ½ cup finely diced red onion

Instructions

- Cook bacon in a small saucepan over medium heat, turning often, until crisp, about 4 minutes. Dran on a paper towel; dcard fat.

- Bring the water and salt to a boil in the pan. Return to a simmer after adding the barley. Reduce heat to low, cover, and simmer for 10 to 12 minutes, or until all of the liquid has been absorbed.

- In a large mixing bowl, combine the hrmmp and lime juice. To coat, add the cooked barley. Allow it stand for 10 minutes, stirring occasionally, to allow the barley to absorb some of the lime juice. Toss in the tomatoes, onion, cilantro, and bacon. Repeat with the oil and pepper. Str in avocado, then serve.

7. Healthy Buddha Bowl Recipes That Will Keep You Satisfied

Ingredients

- 1 medium sweet potato, peeled if desired, cut into 1-inch chunks
- 1 tablespoon lemon juice
- 1 (15 ounces) can 1 15-ounce can chickpeas, rinsed
- ¼ cup chopped fresh cilantro or parsley
- 2 tablespoons tahini
- 2 cups cooked q uinoa
- ½ teaspoon ground pepper, divided
- 1 firm-ripe avocado, diced
- 2 tablespoons water
- ½ teaspoon salt, divided
- 1 small clove garlic, minced
- 3 tablespoons extra-virgin olive oil, divided

Instructions

- Preheat oven to 425 degrees F.

- In a medium bowl, toss sweet potato with 1 tablespoon oil and 1/4 teaspoon each alt and pepper. Transfer to a prepared baking sheet. Roast, turning once, until tender, 15 to 18 minutes.

- In a small dish, combine the remaining 2 tablespoons oil, tahn, water, lemon juice, garlc, and the remaining 1/4 teaspoon each alt and pepper.

- To serve, divide the qiunoa among four bowls. Top with equal parts weet potato, chckpea, and avocado. Drizzle with the tahn auce Sprinkle with parsley (or cilantro).

8. Indian Grain Bowls With Chicken & Vegetables

Ingredients

- 1 cup bulgur

- ½ teaspoon salt

- 1 pound boneless, skinless chicken breasts, trimmed

- 1/2 cup Cilantro Chutney (see Associated Recipes)

- 1 ½ cups water

- 1 cup chopped cucumber

- 1 teaspoon garam masala

- 1 cup sliced grape tomatoes

- 1 cup chopped red bell pepper

- 1 lime, quartered

Instructions

- In a small saucepan, combine bulgur and water; bring to a boil. Reduce heat to low, cover, and simmer for 10 to 15 minutes, or until the bulgur is soft and the liquid has been absorbed. Spread the bulgur on a heet pan to cool before assembling the lunch container.

- Meanwhile, position the rack in the upper third of the oven and preheat the broiler. Coat a broiler pan with cooking spray. Sprnkle checken wth garam maala and alt. Place the chicken on the prepared pan; brol until no longer pink in the centre and an instant-read thermometer inserted into the cake part registers 165 degrees F, 4 to 8 minutes each side. Transfer the chicken to a clean cutting board and let aside for 5 minutes before slicing.

- Transfer 2 tablespoons chutney into each of 4 small lidded containers; refrigerate for up to 4 days.
    - Distribute the cooled bulgur among four ngle-ervng ldded containers. Top each with one-fourth of the chicken and equal amounts of cucumber, bell pepper, and tomato. Each container should have a lime wedge. Seal the container and refrigerate for up to 4 days. Just before serving, top each dish with 1 part of chutney and a squeeze of fresh lime juice to taste.

9. Green Veggie Bowl with Chicken & Lemon-Tahini Dressing

Ingredients

- ¼ cup tahini
- 1 cup 1 small broccoli crown
- ¼ cup lemon juice
- ½ teaspoon minced garlic plus 2 sliced garlic cloves, divided
- ½ large red onion, sliced
- ¼ teaspoon ground pepper
- 1 cup green beans
- ¼ cup chopped fresh cilantro
- 4 (4 ounces) chicken cutlets, trimmed
- ½ teaspoon kosher salt, divided
- 4 cups thinly sliced kale
- ¼ teaspoon ground cumin
- ¼ cup cold water plus 2 tablespoons, divided
- 2 cups cooked brown rice
- 2 tablespoons extra-virgin olive oil, divided

Instructions

- Whisk tahini and 1/4 cup water in a small bowl until smooth. Add lemon juice, minced garlic, cumin, and 1/4 teaspoon salt and whisk to combine. Set aside.

- Trim green beans and cut in half. Break broccoli into florets. Measure 1 cup (reserve the rest for another use).

- Season with the remaining 1/4 teaspoon salt and pepper. 1 tablepoon ol in a large cat-ron kllet over medum heat Cook until an instant-read thermometer registers 160 degrees F, 3 to 5 minutes per side. To stay warm, use a clean cutting board and a tent with fol.

- Wipe out the pan and add the remaining 1 tablespoon of oil. Add onon and cook for 2 minutes, stirring occasionally. Cook for 30 seconds after adding the Iced garlc, then add the broccoli and green beans. Cook, sometimes stirring, for 2 minutes.

Stir in the remaining 2 tablespoons of water. Cover and team for 1 to 2 minutes, or until the veggies are tender-crip.

- Slice the chicken.

- To erve, divide the rice and vegetables into four bowls and top with the chicken. Drizzle with the remaining dressing and sprinkle with cinnamon.

10. Roasted Veggie Brown Rice Buddha Bowl

Ingredients

- 2 tablespoons sliced scallions

- 2 tablespoons chopped fresh cilantro

- 1 cup roasted tofu (see associated recipes)

- ½ cup cooked brown rice (see associated recipes)

- 1 cup roasted vegetables (see associated recipes)

- 2 tablespoons Creamy Vegan Cashew Sauce (see associated recipes)

Instructions

Arrange the rice, vegetables, and tofu in a bowl or 4-cup sealable container. Top with scallions and cilantro. When ready to serve, drizzle with cashew sauce.

11. South Of The Border Buddha Bowl

Ingredients

- 8 ounces extra-firm tofu, cut into 1-inch cubes
- ½ teaspoon chili powder
- ½ cup chopped romaine lettuce
- 1 medium red bell pepper, cut into 1/2-inch strips
- 2 tablespoons toasted pumpkin seeds
- 2 tablespoons lime juice
- ½ avocado
- ⅓ cup of water
- ¼ cup packed cilantro leaves, plus more for garnish
- ½ medium red onion, cut into 1/2-inch wedges
- ½ teaspoon ground coriander
- ¼ teaspoon salt
- 1 tablespoon reduced-sodium tamari or soy sauce
- 1 cup cooked brown rice
- 6 eaches cherry tomatoes, halved
- 5 ⅓ tablespoons 5 tablespoons plus 1 teaspoon extra-virgin olive oil, divided

Instructions

- Preheat oven to 425 degrees F. Line a rimmed baking sheet with parchment paper.

- Tofu, 1 tablespoon oil, tamar (or soy sauce), and cilantro powder in a medium bowl. Place on one half of the prepared baking sheet. To the bowl, add pepper, onon, and 1 teapoon ol; tr to coat. Place the veggies on the other side of the baking sheet. Roast for about 20 minutes, or until the vegetables are tender and the tofu is sizzling.

- Meanwhile, combine the remaining 4 tablespoons of olive oil, avocado, water, cinnamon, lime juice, corander, and salt in a blender jar or mini food processor. Process until smooth, crapping the de as needed.

- Place 1/2 cup rce in each of two salad serving bowls. Top with tofu, roasted vegetables, lettuce, and tomatoes. Spread 4 tablespoons dressing over each bowl and top with pumpkin eed.

12. Vegetarian Sushi Grain Bowl

Ingredients

- 2 cups cooked brown rice
- 2 tablespoons reduced-sodium tamari
- 1 cup shredded carrot
- 1 cup diced cucumber
- 2 teaspoons grated fresh ginger
- 2 tablespoons rice vinegar
- 2 tablespoons avocado oil
- 2 teaspoons toasted (dark) sesame oil
- 1 cup chopped toasted nori
- 1 cup frozen shelled edamame, thawed
- 1 avocado, diced
- 1 teaspoon sesame seeds for garnish

Instructions

Combine rice vinegar, tamari, avocado oil, sesame oil, and ginger in a small bowl.

Distribute brown rce among 4 bowls. Top with equal parts carrot, cucumber, avocado, edamame, and nori. Drizzle with 2 tablespoons dreng each and top with sesame seeds if desired.

13. Rainbow Buddha Bowl With Cashew Tahini Sauce

Ingredients

- 1 tablespoon lemon juice or cider vinegar
- ½ cup cooked quinoa
- ¼ cup sliced cucumber
- ½ cup cooked lentils
- 1 tablespoon extra-virgin olive oil
- ½ teaspoon reduced-sodium tamari or soy sauce (see Tip)
- ¼ teaspoon salt
- ¾ cup unsalted cashews
- ¼ cup chopped bell pepper
- ½ cup shredded red cabbage
- ¼ cup grated raw beet
- ½ cup of water
- ¼ cup grated carrot
- ¼ cup packed parsley leaves
- 1 tablespoon Toasted chopped cashews for garnish

Instructions

- Blend cashews, water, parsley, lemon juice (or vinegar), oil, tamari (or soy sauce), and salt in a blender until smooth.
- Place lentil and quinoa in the centre of a small serving bowl. Top with cabbage, beets, peppers, carrots, and cucumber. Spread 2 tablespoons cashew sauce on top (save the remaining sauce for later use). If desired, garnish with cashews.

Tip: People with celiac disease or gluten sensitivity should use "gluten-free" soy sauce, as soy sauce may include wheat or other gluten-containing sweeteners and flavours.

14. Chickpea & Veggie Grain Bowl

Ingredients

- 1 tablespoon crumbled feta cheese
- ¼ cup canned chickpeas, rinsed
- 1 cup roasted root vegetables (see associated recipes)
- 1 cup mixed salad greens
- 1 cup cooked q uinoa (see associated recipes)

Instructions

- Combine quinoa, greens, roasted vegetables, chickpeas, and feta in a bowl.

15. Vegan Roasted Vegetable Quinoa Bowl With Creamy Green Sauce

Ingredients

- 2 eaches large shallots, sliced
- 2 cups cooked quinoa
- ½ teaspoon salt, divided
- 1 cup shredded red cabbage
- 1 tablespoon cider vinegar
- ¼ teaspoon ground pepper
- 8 ounces cremini mushrooms (3 cups), quartered
- ½ cup of water
- ¼ cup fresh parsley leaves
- 4 cups broccoli florets
- ½ teaspoon reduced-sodium tamari or soy sauce (see Tip)
- ¾ cup raw cashews
- 2 tablespoons extra-virgin olive oil, divided

Instructions

- Preheat oven to 425 degrees F.

- In a large bowl, combine the broccoli, mushrooms, and hallot. Toss in 1 tablespoon of oil, 1/4 teaspoon of salt, and pepper to coat. Transfer to a large rimmed baking sheet and roast, turning once, for about 20 minutes, or until the vegetables are tender and browned.

- In a blender, combine cashews, water, parsley, vinegar, tamar (or oy sauce), and the remaining 1 tablespoon oil and 1/4 teaspoon salt. Puree, toppng, and scraping down the de a need, till mooth.

- Divide cooked q uinoa, cabbage, and the roasted vegetables and sauce among 4 bowls.

Tip: People with celiac disease or gluten sensitivities should use "gluten-free" oil sauces; otherwise, oil sauce may include wheat or other gluten-containing ingredients.

16. Black Bean-Quinoa Buddha Bowl

Ingredients

- ¾ cup canned black beans, rinsed

- 1 tablespoon lime juice

- ¼ cup hummus

- ⅔ cup cooked q uinoa

- 2 tablespoons chopped fresh cilantro

- 3 tablespoons pico de gallo

- ¼ medium avocado, diced

Instructions

In a mixing dish, combine bean and quinoa. Str hummu and lime juice in a small bowl; then add water to desired consistency. Drizzle the hummus over the beans and quinoa. Top with avacado, pico de gallo, and cilantro.

Tips: To make ahead: Assemble the Buddha bowl up to 1 day ahead of time, with the dressing on the side. To prevent avocado browning if making ahead, ueeze an ueeze of lime juice after dcng.

17. Vegan Superfood Buddha Bowls

Ingredients

- 1 cup 1 (8 ounces) pouch microwavable q uinoa

- 1 (5 ounces) package baby kale

- 2 tablespoons lemon juice

- ½ cup hummus

- 1 (15 ounces) can 1 (8 ounces) package refrigerated cooked whole baby beets, sliced (or 2 cups from the salad bar)

- 1 medium avocado, sliced

- 1 cup frozen shelled edamame, thawed
- ¼ cup unsalted toasted sunflower seeds

Instructions

- Prepare q uinoa according to package Instructions: set aside to cool.

- In a small bowl, combine hummus and lemon juice. Then add water to get the required dreng consistency. Distribute the dressing into four small condiment containers and chill.

- Divide the young kale into four single-serving containers with lids. Top each with 1/2 cup unoa, 1/2 cup beet, 1/4 cup edamame, and 1 tablespoon sunflower eed.

- When ready to eat, top with 1/4 avocado and the hummus dressing.

Tips To Make Ahead: Refrigerate bowl and drinking separately for up to 4 days. To avoid bruising, don't add the avocado until you're ready to eat.

18. Jackfruit Barbacoa Burrito Bowls

Ingredients

- 2 tablespoons olive oil
- 6 eaches garlic cloves, crushed
- 1 cup chopped white onion
- 1 medium New Mexico chile, stem and seeds removed
- 1 teaspoon chili powder
- 2 (20 ounce) cans green jackfruit in brine, rinsed and shredded
- 1 lime, q uartered
- ½ teaspoon kosher salt
- 3 cups hot cooked brown rice
- 1 bay leaf
- ½ teaspoon ground pepper
- ½ cup chopped fresh cilantro
- 1 ⅓ cups chopped plum tomatoes (about 3 medium)
- 1 cup unsalted canned black beans, rinsed
- 2 cups thinly sliced iceberg lettuce
- 1 ½ cups unsalted vegetable broth

Instructions

- Heat oil in a medium saucepan over medium-high heat. Cook, stirring occasionally, for approximately 6 minutes, or until the onion is tender and caramelised. Increase the heat to high and bring to a boil. Cover partially and reduce heat to medium. Cook for about 10 minutes, or until the chle is tender. Blend the mixture in a blender. Remove the centre piece of the blender lid (to allow the tea to envelop); replace the top on the blender. Place a clean towel over the opening and proceed until extremely smooth, about 45 seconds. (Be careful while blending hot liquids.)

- Return the chile sauce to the aucepan; stir in the jackfruit, chilli powder, salt, pepper, and bay leaf. Bring to a simmer over medium-high heat. Reduce heat to medium-low, partially cover, and cook until lightly thckened, 6 to 8 minutes.

Remove the bay leaf.

- Place 3/4 cup rce in each of four small bowls. Top with 3/4 cup jackfruit combination, 1/2 cup lettuce, 1/3 cup tomatoes, 1/4 cup bean, and 2 tablespoons cilantro. Serve with slices of lime.

19. Lemon-Roasted Vegetable Hummus Bowls

Ingredients

- 1 ½ cups cauliflower florets
- 1 cup hummus (see Tip)
- ¾ cup diced red bell pepper (1-inch)
- 1 tablespoon extra-virgin olive oil
- 1 medium avocado
- ¼ teaspoon salt
- 2 cloves garlic, thinly sliced
- ¾ cup diced zucchini (1-inch) 2 teaspoons lemon zest
- 2 cups cooked tricolor quinoa, cooled
- 1 ½ cups broccoli florets
- 4 wedge (blank)s lemon wedges
- 1 teaspoon dried oregano

Instructions

- Preheat the oven to 425°F. Combine cauliflower, broccoli, and garlic on an rmmed baking sheet. Drizzle with oil and sprinkle with oregano and salt; stir to coat. 10 minutes in the oven

- Stir in the bell pepper and zucchini to the vegetables in the pan. Roast for 10 to 15 minutes more, or until the veggies are crisp-tender and gently browned. Sprnkle lemon zet over the vegetable; ade to cool before aemblng bowl.

- Distribute the roasted vegetables among four single-serving containers. Add a lemon wedge to each container and top with 1/2 cup unoa and 1/4 cup hummu. Refrigerate for up to 4 days after sealing the containers. To serve, squeeze the lemon wedge over the bowl and top with one-fourth diced avocado.

20. Crispy Chickpea Grain Bowl With Lemon Vinaigrette

Ingredients

- ¼ teaspoon ground pepper, divided
- 1 ⅓ cups water plus 1 tablespoon, divided
- ⅔ cup quinoa
- 1 (15 ounces) can no-salt-added chickpeas, rinsed
- 2 tablespoons toasted pumpkin seeds
- 2 teaspoons lemon zest
- ⅛ teaspoon salt plus 1/4 teaspoon, divided
- 1 teaspoon Dijon mustard
- 2 tablespoons lemon juice
- 1 clove garlic, minced
- ¼ cup crumbled feta cheese
- 1 bunch kale, stems removed, thinly sliced (about 5 cups)
- 1 red bell pepper, thinly sliced
- 4 teaspoons extra-virgin olive oil plus 2 tablespoons, divided
- 1 small red onion, thinly sliced

Instructions

- Preheat oven to 400 degrees F. Coat a large rimmed baking sheet liberally with cooking spray.

- In a medium saucepan, combine quinoa, 1 1/3 cups water, and 1/8 teaspoon salt. Bring to a boil over medium-high heat. Reduce the heat to medium-low, partially cover, and simmer for 15 minutes, or until the quinoa tender. Drain any excess water.

- Meanwhile, dry chckpeas with a paper towel. In a large bowl, combine one onion, two tablespoons of oil, and one-eighth teaspoon of salt and pepper. Spread on the prepared baking sheet. Cook for 15 minutes.

- Tos kale with 2 teapots of oil and the remaining 1/8 teapot of salt in a big dish. Stir in the kale and continue to roast for 15 minutes.

- In a small bowl, combine mustard, garlic, lemon zest, lemon juice, the remaining 1 tablespoon water, and the remaining 1/8 teaspoon pepper. Stir in the remaining 2 tablespoons of oil.
- Divide the quinoa among 4 serving bowls. Top with the kale mixture, bell pepper slices, feta, and pumpkin seeds. Drizzle with the vinaigrette.

21. Oatmeal-Rhubarb Porridge

Ingredients

- 2 tablespoons chopped pecans or other nuts, toasted.

- ½ teaspoon ground cinnamon

- 1 cup old-fashioned rolled oats

- 1 cup 1/2-inch pieces rhubarb, fresh or frozen

- 1 pinch Pinch of salt

- ½ cup of orange juice

- 3 tablespoons 2-3 tablespoons brown sugar, pure maple syrup or agave syrup

- 1 ½ cups 1 1/2 cups nonfat milk or nondairy milk, such as soymilk or almond milk

Instructions

- In a medium aucepan, combine milk, juice, oatmeal, rhubarb, cinnamon, and salt. Bring to a boil on medium-high heat. Reduce the heat to low, cover, and simmer for 5 minutes, stirring often, until the oatmeal and rhubarb are soft. Remove from the heat and leave covered for 5 minutes. Add weetener to taste. Finish with nuts.

Tip: To toast chopped nuts, place them in a small dry kllet and cook over medium-low heat, turning constantly, until crisp and lightly browned, 2 to 4 minutes. People with celiac disease or gluten intolerance should consume "gluten-free" oats, as oats are frequently cross-contaminated with wheat and barley.

21. Amaranth Pudding With Amaretto Cream

Ingredients

- 1 3-inch cinnamon stick
- ¾ cup nonfat milk
- 2 tablespoons amaretto l iq ueur
- ¾ cup half-and-half
- ¼ teaspoon salt
- ¼ tablespoon 1/4 cup plus 2 tablespoons turbinado sugar
- 3 ½ cups 3-3 1/2 cups water
- 1 teaspoon vanilla extract
- 1 ½ cups 1 1/2 cups amaranth (see Tips)

Amaretto Cream &Amp; Topping

- ½ cup whipping cream
- 16 eaches amaretti cookies, divided
- 2 teaspoons amaretto liqueur, plus more for drizzle
- 1 tablespoon confectioners sugar

Instructions

To make the pudding, combine 3 cups water, amaranth, and cinnamon powder in a large heavy saucepan; bring to a boil over medium-high heat, stirring occasionally with a wooden spoon. Reduce heat to maintain a simmer, cover, and cook, stirring occasionally, until thickened and the amaranth tender and tranlucent, 18 to 20 minutes. If the amaranth begins to stick to the bottom of the pan, add 1/4 to 1/2 cup more water. Dcard the cnnamon tck.

Str in half-and-half, milk, turbnado sugar, 2 tablespoons amaretto, vanlla, and alt; return to a mmer, trrrng constantly. Reduce heat to maintain a moderate bubble and cook, stirring constantly, until the mixture resembles a thick porridge, 3 to 5 minutes more. Reduce heat more if necessary to prevent puddles from forming on the pan. (Use cauton a you tr: the mxture can platter a you tr.) Divide the pudding across 8 small serving dishes (about 2/3 cup each). Allow to cool at room temperature for 1 hour. Cover with plastic wrap and refrigerate until chilled, at least 1 hour.

To prepare the amaretti cream and topping: When preparing to erve, whip cream, confectioners' ugar, and 2 teapoon amaretto in a medium bowl with a electrc mxer on medium peed until oft peak form. Using your fingers, cruh 8 cook to get crumbs. Top each puddle with about 1 tablespoon whipped cream and 1 tablespoon cooked crumb. Garnish each bowl with 1 whole cook and a drizzle of amaretto, if preferred.

Make-Ahead Tip: Prepare the pudding (Steps 1 & 2) up to 2 days ahead of time.

Tips: Amaranth, which is high in protein and minerals like calcium and magnesium, has been farmed in Central America for an estimated 5,000 to 8,000 years. When cooked, it has a thick, porridge-like texture that is great in soups, tew, morning porridge, or pudding. It can be found in the natural-food department of a well-stocked supermarket or natural-food store.

To Make It Gluten-Free: Most Italian almond cookies are prepared without gluten-containing ingredients, however not all brands are made in a gluten-free facility. If you are gluten-free, use almond-flavored gluten-free cookies for the topping.

22. Bacony Barley Salad With Marinated Shrimp

Ingredients

- 3 piece (blank)s 3 strips bacon, chopped

- ⅔ cup q uick-cooking barley

- ½ teaspoon salt

- 1 ⅓ cups water

- 2 cups cherry tomatoes, halved

- ⅓ cup lime juice

- 1 pound peeled cooked shrimp, (21-25 per pound; thawed if frozen), tails removed, coarsely chopped

- 2 tablespoons extra-virgin olive oil

- ½ cup chopped fresh cilantro

- ½ cup finely diced red onion

- 1 avocado, peeled and diced

- 1 Freshly ground pepper, to taste

Instructions

- Cook bacon in a small saucepan over medium heat, turning often, until crisp, about 4 minutes. Drain on a paper towel and discard the fat.

- Bring the water and salt to a boil in a saucepan. Return to a summer after adding barley. Reduce heat to low, cover, and mmer for 10 to 12 minutes, or until all the liquid has been absorbed.

- Combine hrmp and lime juice in a large bowl. Toss in the cooked barley to coat. Allow the barley to absorb some of the lime juice by standing for 10 minutes and occasionally turning. To coat, add the tomatoes, onion, cilantro, and bacon. Add ol and pepper and stir one more. Strn avocado and serve

Make-Ahead Tip: Prepare without avocado, cover, and refrigerate for up to 2 days. Stir in the avocado just before serving.

23. Sesame-Honey Tempeh & Quinoa Bowl

Ingredients

Quinoa &Amp; Carrot Slaw

- 1 ½ cups water

- 2 tablespoons rice vinegar

- 1 tablespoon sesame oil

- 1 tablespoon reduced-sodium soy sauce

- 2 tablespoons sesame seeds, toasted (see Tip)

- 2 cups grated carrots (about 3 large)
- ¾ cup q uinoa, rinsed

Sesame-Honey Tempeh

- 3 tablespoons honey

- 2 ounces 2 8-ounce packages tempeh (see Note), crumbled into bite-size pieces

- 2 tablespoons sesame oil

- 2 eaches scallions, sliced

- 1 teaspoon cornstarch

- 2 tablespoons water

- 3 tablespoons reduced-sodium soy sauce

Instructions

- To prepare unoa: Bring 1 1/2 cups water to a boil in a small aucepan. Return to a bol after adding unoa. Reduce to a low simmer, cover, and cook for 10 to 14 minutes, or until the water has been absorbed. Uncover and let stand.

- To make carrot law: Meanwhile, in a medium bowl, add carrots, rice vinegar, sesame seeds, 1 tablespoon oil, and 1 tablespoon soy sauce. Set aside.

- To make tempeh, heat 2 tablespoons oil in a large nonstick skillet over medium heat. Cook, stirring often, until the tempeh begins to brown, 7 to 9 minutes.

- In a small bowl, combine honey, 3 tablespoons oy auce, 2 tablespoons water, and cornstarch. Cook, stirring constantly, until the sauce thickens and coats the tempeh, about 1 minute.

- Divide the unoa into four bowls and top each with 1/2 cup carrot lettuce and 3/4 cup tempeh mixture. Garnish with onions.

Tip: To toast the same eed, set it in a small dry pan and cook over medium-low heat, stirring regularly, until fragrant and lightly browned, 2 to 4 minutes.

24. Whole-Grain Pizza Dough

Ingredients

- ½ teaspoon salt
- 1 ¼ cups bread flour or all-purpose flour
- 1 teaspoon sugar
- 1 teaspoon instant or RapidRise yeast
- ¾ cup 3/4 cup white whole-wheat flour (see Tips) or all-purpose flour
- ⅔ cup lukewarm water

Instructions

Str water, yeat, and ugar n a large bowl; let tand for 5 mnute till the yeat has dolved. Str n bread flour (or all-PURPOSE flour), whole-wheat flour (or all-PURPOSE flour), and alt till the dough comes together.

Turn out the dough onto a lightly floured work surface. Knead for about 10 minutes, or until the dough is smooth and elastic. (Alternatively, you may combine the dough in a food processor.) Process until it forms a ball, then knead for 1 minute.) Pour the dough into a oled basin and turn to coat.

Cover the basin with a clean kitchen towel and set aside in a warm, draft-free location for about 1 hour, or until the dough has about doubled in size.

Make-Ahead Tip: Prepare to Step 2, then cover the bowl with plastic wrap and chill for up to 1 day. Alternatively, securely wrap the unren dough in oiled plastic wrap and freeze for up to 3 months. Overnight defrost in the refrigerator. Let it be refrigerated (or previously frozen).

Storage Smarts: Wrap your food in a layer of plastic wrap followed by a layer of foil for long-term freezer storage. The platic will help avoid freezer burn, while the flour will help prevent off-odor from evaporating into the food.

25. Toasted Quinoa Salad With Scallops & Snow Peas

Ingredients

- 2 teaspoons grated or minced garlic
- 12 ounces dry sea scallops, cut into 1/2-inch pieces, or dry bay scallops (see Note)
- 4 teaspoons 4 tablespoons plus 2 teaspoons canola oil, divided
- 1 ½ cups 1 1/2 cups q uinoa, rinsed well (see Tip)
- 4 teaspoons reduced-sodium tamari, or soy sauce, divided
- ⅓ cup of rice vinegar
- 1 teaspoon salt
- 1 cup trimmed and diagonally sliced snow peas, (1/2 inch thick)
- ¼ cup 1/4 cup finely chopped fresh cilantro, for garnish
- ⅓ cup finely diced red bell pepper
- 1 teaspoon toasted sesame oil
- 1 cup thinly sliced scallions
- 3 cups of water

Instructions

- Toss scallops with 2 teaspoons tamari (or soy sauce) in a medium bowl. Set aside.
- Heat a big, high-sided skillet with a tight-fitting cover over medium heat. 1 tablespoon canola oil and 1 teaspoon qiunoa Cook, stirring constantly, for 6 to 8 minutes, or until the unoa begins to colour. Cook, stirring constantly, until fragrant, about 1 minute more. Bring the water and salt to a boil. Cook over medium heat for about 15 minutes, or until the water is absorbed. (Do not tr.) Remove from the heat and let aside for 5 minutes, covered. Stir in the peas, cover, and let aside for another 5 minutes.
- In a large bowl, combine 3 tablespoons canola oil, the remaining 2 teaspoons tamar (or oy auce), vnegar, and eame oil. Toss in the unoa and snow peas, scallions, and bell pepper to combine.
- Take the scallops out of the marinade and blot them dry. Heat a large kettle over medium heat until it is hot enough to evaporate a drop of water on contact. Add the remaining 2 teapoon canola ol and cook, turning once, until golden and barely

frm, about 2 minutes total. tr the callop nto the unoa alad gently. If desired, garnish with cilantro.

Note: Buy "dry" callop, which is callop that has not been treated with odum trpolyphophate or STP. STP-treated scallops ("wet" scallops) have been exposed to a chemical bath and are mushy, less delicious, and will not brown correctly.

Tip: Quinoa is a flavorful, protein-rich grain. Rinsing removes all traces of aponn, unoa's natural, protective coating. It may be found at natural-food stores and the natural-foods section of many supermarkets. People with celiac disease or gluten intolerance should use soy sauce labelled "gluten-free," as soy sauce may include wheat or other gluten-containing sweetener and flavouring.

26. Barley Hoppin' John

Ingredients

- 1 tablespoon extra-virgin olive oil
- 1 small red bell pepper, chopped
- 1 medium onion, chopped
- ¼ teaspoon crushed red pepper
- 2 cloves garlic, minced
- 1 (14.1 ounces) can 1 14-ounce can vegetable broth
- 2 teaspoons lemon juice
- 1 tablespoon chopped fresh thyme or 1 teaspoon dried
- 2 eaches 2 stalks celery, chopped
- 1 cup quick-cooking barley
- ¼ teaspoon salt
- 2 (15 ounce) cans 2 15-ounce cans black-eyed peas, rinsed

Instructions

- Heat the oil in a large nonstick kettle over medium heat. Add the onion, bell pepper, and celery. Cook for 3 to 4 minutes, or until the vegetables are tender. Cook for 1 minute after adding garlic. Add the broth, barley, thyme, lemon juice, crushed red pepper, and salt and bring to a boil. Reduce heat, cover, and simmer for 15 to 20 minutes, or until the barley is done. Remove from the heat and mix in the black-eyed pea. Cover and stand for 5 minutes. Serve warm.

27. Lemongrass Pork & Spaghetti Sq uash Noodle Bowl with Peanut Sauce

Ingredients

- 2 tablespoons light brown sugar
- 2 tablespoons minced fresh lemongrass (see Tip)
- 2 tablespoons minced fresh ginger, divided
- 2 tablespoons reduced-sodium soy sauce
- 1 pound baby spinach
- 1 tablespoon fish sauce
- 1 pound 1 2 1/2- to 3-pound spaghetti sq uash, halved lengthwise and seeded
- 3 tablespoons peanut oil, divided
- 1 pound pork tenderloin, cut into 1/2-inch slices
- ¼ cup smooth natural peanut butter
- ½ cup "lite" coconut milk
- ¼ cup of water

Instructions

- In a hallow dish, combine 1 tablespoon ginger, lemongra, brown ugar, soy sauce, and fish sauce. Add the pork, flip to coat, and set aside for 20 minutes, turning once or twice.

- Meanwhile, place s uah cut-de down n a mcrowave-afe dh; add 2 tablepoon water. Microwave on High for 10 minutes, or until the fleh is soft. (Alternatively, place uah halve cut-side down on a rimmed baking sheet.) Bake at 400°F for 40 to 50 minutes, or until the uah tender.)

- In a big skillet, heat 2 tablepoon ol over medium-high heat. Add the remaining 1 tablespoon gnger and a few handfuls of spinach at a time, cooking and stirring until all of the spinach has wilted, 1 to 2 minutes total. Transfer to a platter and cover to keep heated.

- Wipe out the pan, add the remaining 1 tablespoon of oil, and heat on medium-high. Cook, turning once, until the pork (and marinade) is browned, about 2 minutes per side. Transfer the pork to the pan with the sauce and cover; leave the liquid in the pan.

- Add coconut milk, peanut butter, and 1/4 cup water to the pan; cook for 1 minute, stirring and scraping off any brown bits.
- To serve, scrape the uah from the hell with a fork and distribute it among four bowls. Drizzle each porton with 2 tablespoons peanut sauce, then top with pork and pnach, then drizzle with the remaining peanut sauce.

Tips

Find lemongra—a woody, callon-shaped herb with an aromatic lemon flavor—in the produce section of well-stocked supermarkets or Asian food markets. To use, trim the root end and grey top. Remove the outer layer and just Ice (or mnce) the softer inner talk.

Cut Down On Dishes: A rimmed baking sheet is ideal for anything from roasting to catching inadvertent drips and pll. Line your baking sheets with foil before each use for easy cleanup and to keep them in tip-top shape.

28. Mediterranean Chicken Quinoa Bowl

Ingredients

- 1-pound boneless, skinless chicken breasts, trimmed
- 4 tablespoons extra-virgin olive oil, divided
- ¼ teaspoon ground pepper
- 1 small clove garlic, crushed
- ¼ cup slivered almonds
- ¼ teaspoon salt
- 7 ounces 1 7-ounce jar roasted red peppers, rinsed
- ¼ teaspoon crushed red pepper
- ½ teaspoon ground cumin
- 1 teaspoon paprika
- 2 cups cooked quinoa
- ¼ cup pitted Kalamata olives, chopped
- 1 cup diced cucumber
- ¼ cup finely chopped red onion
- 2 tablespoons finely chopped fresh parsley
- ¼ cup crumbled feta cheese

Instructions

- Position a rack in the upper third of the oven; preheat broiler to high. Line a rimmed baking sheet with foil.

- Sprinkle the chicken with salt and pepper and place it on the prepared baking sheet. Cook for 14 to 18 minutes, or until an instant-read thermometer inserted in the thickest part reads 165 degrees Fahrenheit. Place the chicken on a clean cutting board and Ice or hred.

- Meanwhile, in a mixing bowl, combine the peppers, almonds, 2 tablespoons oil, garlic, paprika, cumin, and crushed red pepper (if using). Purée until completely smooth.

- Combine quinoa, olives, red onion, and the remaining 2 tablespoons oil in a medium bowl.
- To serve, divide the quinoa mixture among four bowls and top with equal portions of cucumber, chicken, and red pepper sauce. Sprinkle with feta and parsley.

Make-Ahead Tip: Prepare the chicken (Step 2), red pepper sauce (Step 3), and unoa (Step 4); refrigerate in a separate container. Just before serving, assemble.

29. Turmeric Rice Bowl with Garam Masala Root Vegetables & Chickpeas

Ingredients

Rice

- 1 ¼ cups water
- ⅛ teaspoon kosher salt
- 1 teaspoon onion powder or garlic powder
- 1 teaspoon extra-virgin olive oil
- ¼ cup raisins
- ¼ teaspoon ground black pepper grated turmeric
- ¼ teaspoon ground cinnamon
- ½ teaspoon ground turmeric or 1 teaspoon freshly
- ½ cup brown basmati rice

Vegetables &Amp; Chickpeas

- Chopped fresh herbs, such as mint, parsley, and/or cilantro, for garnish
- 2 tablespoons lemon juice
- 1 teaspoon garam masala or Indian curry powder
- 1 (15 ounces) can chickpeas, rinsed and patted dry
- 1 teaspoon sugar or honey
- ¼ teaspoon kosher salt
- ¼ teaspoon ground pepper
- 1 cup roasted root vegetables (see associated recipe)
- plain yogurt or tahini 2 tablespoons low-fat
- 2 tablespoons coconut oil or ghee

Instructions

- To make rce, combine water, rce, ran, olive oil, on powder (or garlc powder), turmerc, cinnamon, pepper, and 1/8 teaspoon tea in a small aucepan. Bring the water to a boil. Cover, lower heat to a gentle simmer, and cook for 35 to 40 minutes, or until the liquid is absorbed. Remove from the heat and let aside for 10 minutes, covered.

- To prepare veggies & chckpea, heat coconut ol (or ghee) in a medium kettle over medium heat. Cook, stirring constantly, until the chickpeas are crispy, 3 to 5 minutes. Stir in garam masala (or curry powder) and cook until fragrant, about 1 minute. Add roasted root vegetables, ugar (or honey), salt, and pepper; cook, stirring often, until cooked through, 2 to 4 minutes. Stir in the lemon juice.
- Serve the vegetable mixture over the rice, topped with yogurt (or tahini). Garnish with herbs, if desired.

30. Roasted Eggplant, Zucchini & Pork Bowls

IngredientsQuinoa & Salad

- 1 ¼ cups water

- 1 small eggplant (10-12 ounces), cut into 1/2-inch cubes

- 1 pound lean ground pork

- 1 teaspoon extra-virgin olive oil plus 2 tablespoons, divided

- ½ cup finely chopped fresh cilantro

- ¾ cup quinoa

- ½ teaspoon salt

- 1-pint cherry tomatoes

- 1 medium zucchini, cut into 1/2-inch cubes

Miso Sauce

- 2 tablespoons white miso (see Tips)

- 3 tablespoons water

- 1 teaspoon grated fresh ginger

- 1 medium garlic, minced

- 1 tablespoon toasted (dark) sesame oil

- 1 ½ tablespoons tahini (see Tips)
- 2 tablespoons rice vinegar

Instructions

- **To Prepare Quinoa:** Bring water and qiunoa to a boil in a small aucepan. Reduce the heat, cover, and mmer for about 15 minutes, or until the water is absorbed. Remove from the heat and let aside for 5 minutes. Str n clantro.

- **To Prepare Sauce:** Whisk water, mo, vinegar, tahini, seaame oil, garlic, and ginger in a small bowl until smooth. Set aside.

- **To Prepare Salad:** In a 14-nch flat-bottom wok, heat 1 teapoon olve ol over medium-high heat. Cook, stirring occasionally, until the meat is cooked through, 5 to 7 minutes. Refer to a plate. Add the remaining 2 tablespoons oil, eggplant, zucchini, tomatoes, and salt to the pan and cook, turning occasionally, until the veggies are soft, 6 to 8 minutes. Return the pork to the pan and swirl to combine.

- Divide the qiunoa into four bowls and top with the pork mxture. Drizzle each serving with a generous 2 tablespoons of miso sauce.

Some people believe that the Dr. Seb food list is too long for them. However, faithful adherents of the diet believe that there is enough food on the list to provide for variety. A typical Dr. Seb diet dinner can include vegetables sautéed in avocado oil on a bed of wild rice, or a large green salad with an olive oil vinaigrette and a sprinkle of agave yrup. Although it may take some getting accustomed to, Dr. Sebi's food list may be simple to follow and beneficial to one's health.

Welcome to a new way of eating and living. This cookbook was created just for your transition from eating man-made to eating God-given food. Consider it a journey. It is not always easy to stop eating the many acidic foods that we have grown accustomed to - but it is possible to do so by cleaning and replenishing our bodies with the food that the Creator has supplied. These recipes reflect years of healing and sharing by our clients, friends, and coworkers. Relax and enjoy the ride.

Dr. Seb' det received no centfc research support. However, it may provide some of the advantages associated with other plant-based diets. Eating more whole fruits and vegetables may have a positive impact on health. It might also assist a person lose weight if that is a goal. The Dr. Seb diet, on the other hand, might pose hazards. It is critical to ensure that the body is getting enough nutrients, including vitamin B-12, through supplementation if necessary.

Certain people may be particularly vulnerable to the hazards associated with the Dr. Seb diet. Adolescents, women who are nursing, and elderly adults are among them.

The diet's proponents recommend pricey products with no scientific evidence to back them up. A more healthful approach may be to eat more plant-based foods and to supplement any missing nutrients. Before attempting any new diet, conduct research and contact with a health care professional.

BOOK 12
Doctor Sebi's Cure for Herpes

How to Cure Herpes Simplex Virus with Dr. Sebi's Alkaline diet

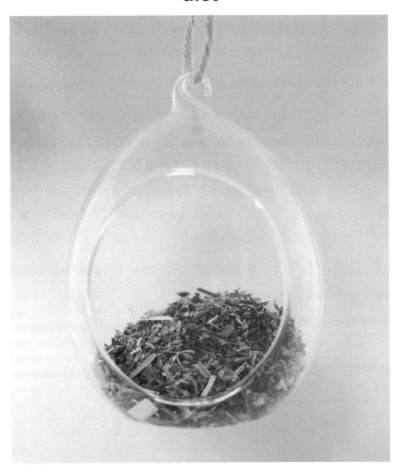

A sexually transmitted illness that is common and has been around for millions of years is herpes simplex virus (HSV). The presence of this virus in the human body system can cause various illnesses, from minor skin and mucous membrane conditions to more serious conditions that disrupt the central nervous system (CNS) and may ultimately result in death, particularly in patients with weakened immune systems. Patients with the herpes simplex virus condition needing treatment are common for doctors who specialize in many areas of medicine.

The late Dr. Sebi created Dr. Sebi's alkaline diet, a plant-based eating plan, to aid in cell renewal and maintain the pH of the body's system. This is done by alkalizing the blood by removing toxic waste from the body. This alkaline diet focuses on consuming a select group of foods listed together with several supplements.

Dr. Sebi created this diet to promote the body's general health without the need for western pharmaceuticals, not just for naturally treating and avoiding diseases.

Dr. Sebi found that the accumulation of mucus in a body part or organ causes sickness. For instance, too much phlegm in the pancreas causes diabetes, whereas too much mucus in the lungs causes pneumonia. He thoroughly lists the fruits, vegetables, cereals, seeds, nuts, herbs, and oils that are best for an alkaline diet. Additionally, using animal products is not permitted; the Dr. Sebi diet is regarded as a vegan diet.

Is Herpes Simplex Virus Entirely a Sexually Transmitted Disease?

Both sexual and non-sexual methods can be used to spread the herpes simplex virus. Herpes simplex virus type 1 is usually oral herpes since it is primarily acquired through oral contact. By sharing a cup of liquid with an infected individual, kissing them, or making any other sort of lip contact with them, you run the risk of getting the virus. Herpes simplex virus-2 can only be acquired through the genital organs. Thus anyone who engages in sexual activity runs the risk of contracting it.

The Dr. Sebi alkaline diet is a suggested treatment for you if you notice signs of the herpes simplex virus, which can be self-detected.

Dr. Sebi Beliefs and Fundamentals

The alkaline diet recommended by Dr. Sebi includes a variety of nutrients that he also developed and discovered. His diet strongly emphasizes eating foods and using supplements that make the body more alkaline, reducing disease-causing mucous. The six foundational ideas that Dr. Sebi categorized are stated below.

According to Dr. Sebi, there are six basic food groups:

- Live
- Raw
- Dead
- Hybrid
- Genetically modified
- Drugs.

Dr. Sebi's diet eliminates all food groups save for life and raw foods and encourages followers to adhere as closely as possible to a raw vegan diet. Whole grains, fruits, and vegetables are grown naturally are among these foods.

Dr. Sebi described raw foods as "electric," capable of combating the body's acidic food waste. The Dr. Sebi Electric Food List is a list of foods Dr. Sebi developed and believed to be ideal for his diet. Despite Dr. Sebi's passing, the range of Dr. Sebi's products keeps expanding and changing.

It can be difficult to strictly adhere to Dr. Sebi's diet and the Dr. Sebi Food List, especially if you frequently eat out. You need to get used to cooking many vegan meals at home with products like wild rice, agave syrup, olive oil, etc., to follow it wisely.

Types of Herpes Simplex Virus and Its Symptoms

There are primarily two forms of herpes; patients with herpes can be diagnosed with either type (HSV-1) or type (HSV-2) of the herpes simplex virus. The symptoms and methods of transmission of these two forms of herpes vary. HSV-1 is mostly spread by oral contact with an infected person, which results in an infection of the mouth or surrounding areas (oral herpes). HSV-1, on the other hand, can be acquired through oral to-genital contact and cause illness in or near the genital area (genital herpes).

HSV-2 infection in the vaginal or anal region is most often caused by genital-to-genital contact during sex (genital herpes).

Oral herpes infections of both types are practically never diagnosed until they reach a severe level, while genital herpes infections are frequently overlooked. Blisters, boils, and itching in the pubic region are a few possible signs.

Herpes simplex virus type 1 (HSV-1)

HSV-1 is a highly contagious STI that is widespread and endemic worldwide. Most people with HSV-1 infections contracted them as children, and the illness is more difficult to treat. Oral herpes, also known as orolabial herpes, affects about 70% of people with HSV-1 disorders, while genital herpes affects between 30% and 40% of people with HSV-1 diseases (infections in the genital or anal area).

Signs and symptoms

Because oral herpes is asymptomatic, most sufferers are unaware they have the condition. In other words, when it is encountered, the symptoms are not immediately apparent. Hurting blisters or open sores called ulcers in or around the mouth are some signs of oral herpes. The sores on the lips are frequently referred to as "cold sores," and the infected person may most likely experience tingling, stinging, or burning before the lesions form. Usually, the blisters and ulcers appear after the initial infection. Depending on the patient's body system, the virus develops differently.

Due to HSV-1's asymptomatic nature, genital herpes in a person's body system may go unnoticed or only manifest as mild symptoms. The signs of genital herpes include anal and genital sores or ulcers. A patient who has previously had treatment for genital herpes may experience relapses. Although, unlike herpes simplex virus type 2-related genital herpes, HSV-1-caused genital herpes normally does not frequently recur.

Transmission

Herpes simplex virus type 1 is mostly transmitted by oral-to-oral contact, which results in the development of oral herpes through contact with sores, saliva, and surfaces in or near the mouth. Furthermore, oral contact with the vaginal region can spread HSV-1 to the genital area, resulting in genital herpes.

HSV-1 can still spread even if there are no symptoms and the skin and oral surfaces look healthy. Furthermore, when the sore is noticeable and active, there is a higher risk of transmission. HSV-1 genital herpes may not be contracted by patients with HSV-1 oral herpes. Rarely a mother's HSV-1 genital herpes infection can be passed on to her unborn child after childbirth, leading to neonatal herpes.

Possible complications

Patients with weakened immune systems, including HIV patients, may experience more severe symptoms and consequences. Rarely, HSV-1 can cause serious illnesses including encephalitis or keratitis (eye infection) (brain infections).

Neonatal herpes

If the mother has HSV, the infant may contract neonatal herpes during delivery in the mother's vaginal area (HSV-1 or HSV-2). Neonatal herpes is a rare but serious illness that can cause permanent brain damage or death. According to estimates, 1 in 10,000 pregnancies results in a newborn with herpes.

A mother's risk of passing on herpes to her unborn child is low if she had genital herpes before conception. When a mother catches HSV for the first time in late pregnancy, the risk of neonatal herpes is particularly high, in part because the concentration of HSV in the vaginal tract is highest early in an infection.

Herpes simplex virus type 2 (HSV-2)

HSV-2 infection, which causes genital herpes and is quite common worldwide, is nearly exclusively sexually transmitted. HSV-2 is a lifelong, incurable condition. It is a primary contributor to genital herpes, which can also be brought on by type 1 herpes simplex virus (HSV-1). HSV-2-induced genital herpes is a widespread infection. According to estimates, (13%) of people in the world between the ages of 15 and 49 had the condition in 2006, with more women than males affected. The explanation for this is that men are more likely than women to sexually transmit herpes to one another.

Signs and symptoms

Often, there are no symptoms at all in the early stages of genital herpes infections, or there may be minor symptoms that go unnoticed. Due to this, most afflicted individuals are unaware they have the illness. In general, 10–20% of those with HSV-2 infection have had a genital herpes diagnosis in the past. Depending on their bodily system and mechanism, some people may experience HSV-2 symptoms in the early stages.

Genital or anal blisters and open sores, known as ulcers, are the signs of genital herpes. In its early stages, genital herpes can cause fever, swollen lymph nodes, and body aches. People with HSV-2 may suffer shooting pain in the legs, hips, and buttocks, as well as a feeling of mild tingling in these areas before developing genital ulcers.

HSV-2 is mostly spread through sexual activity, bodily secretions, and open wounds. Rarely can a mother's HSV-2 infection pass from her to her baby during birth, resulting in neonatal herpes?

Possible complications

HIV and HSV-2

It has been found that HSV-2 and HIV interact significantly. A patient who has an HSV-2 infection is three times more likely to develop a new HIV infection. Additionally, those who have both HIV and HSV-2 infection are more likely to transmit HIV to others. One of the most prevalent diseases in HIV patients is HSV-2, which affects 60 to 90% of those with the virus.

HSV-2 can cause more serious, albeit uncommon, problems, including retinal necrosis, meningoencephalitis, hepatitis, esophagitis, pneumonitis, or widespread infection in those with advanced HIV diseases.

A New Way to Treat Herpes

Be aware that HSV is a viral illness, and currently, no recognized treatment exists. The precaution is to treat the symptoms or significantly lessen them. Even after the symptoms have subsided, the virus is still present. The symptoms could return if the right treatments are not taken.

With a mix of lifestyle adjustments, food modifications, and supplementation, you will unquestionably be able to lower inflammation, irritation, and other symptoms. During his lifetime, Dr. Sebi identified several crucial diets, herbal remedies, and supplements for correctly managing the most difficult-to-treat illnesses, HSV included. Simple fruits and herbs that you may find nearby are used in these tried-and-true natural diets and medicines to help reduce swellings, stinging, and itching.

Is Dr. Sebi's Herpes Cure Effective?

According to Dr. Sebi's study, inflammation can occur when the blood's alkalinity is altered, and the body's system is excessively acidic, making it unable to fight against illnesses and diseases. Many people have reported success with Dr. Sebi's alkaline diet, which has also reportedly helped others eliminate all HSV symptoms in their bodies.

You will cleanse and return your body to its natural alkaline condition by faithfully adhering to his dietary and supplement recommendations. Dr. Sebi maintains that for your body to cure itself, you must wisely adhere to the diet for the rest of your life.

Due to the low protein content of this diet, no beans, lentils, or soy products are included.

Different supplements that quickly cleanse and rejuvenate the body make up Dr. Sebi's supplements, which claim to nourish your cells while purifying your body.

Customers are strongly encouraged to purchase the "all-inclusive" package, which includes 20 different purportedly cleansing goods.

The eight guidelines for Dr. Sebi's diet must be followed. They emphasize staying away from ultra-processed meals and animal products. The diet recommends consuming just natural foods rather than an exotic diet heavy in ultra-processed foods high in salt, sugar, fat, and calories.

Potential benefits of the Dr. Sebi diet:

- It heavily emphasizes meals that come from plants.

- The diet promotes consuming a lot of fiber, vitamins, minerals, and plant chemicals.

- Because certain fruits and vegetables contain substances that make it easier for users to obtain other diseases and prevent them from acquiring them, inflammation and oxidative stress are significantly decreased.

- Additionally, a large part of Dr. Sebi's diet consists of whole grains high in fiber and healthy fats, including nuts, seeds, and plant oils. These foods make it harder to get herpes and make it easier for it to recover.

- The only high-calorie foods in Dr. Sebi's diet are avocados, seeds, and oils. Except for nuts, seeds, avocados, and oils, most items on this diet have few calories, even when you consume a lot of them. Therefore, there is little possibility of becoming obese even when it is ingested in huge amounts.

- Dr. Sebi's diet strongly focuses on consuming nutrient-dense produce, whole grains, and healthy fats, which may reduce inflammation and the risk of developing additional diseases.

Dr. Sebi's Approach to a Herpes Cure

According to Dr. Sebi's study, illnesses and infections cannot exist in an alkaline environment. Hence a high blood alkalinity level is necessary to prevent the body from contracting herpes. It is essential to consume an electrolyte-rich diet to maintain the body's alkalinity and strengthen the immune system. Combining a few lifestyle adjustments listed below, the initial approach to HSV is to lessen inflammations, irritations, sores, and other symptoms.

- Warm compresses — Using heat to relieve the discomfort of sores that are developing or have already developed can help to significantly lessen the swellings. A half-filled rice sock may be microwaved for 40 to 1 minute to create a dry, warm compress.

- Compressing cool air can also help to reduce edema. Apply an ice pack or a clean washcloth loaded with ice to the swollen region. Apply after every four hours.

- Baking soda paste: This aids in drying up sores and alleviating irritation. To apply this, dab a damp cotton ball on the afflicted region after dipping it into a tiny amount of pure baking soda.

- The paste made of corn starch - Paste made of corn starch can also be used to dry up lesions and reduce irritation. Apply cornstarch to the wound by dipping a damp cotton ball or Q-tip into the substance.

- Topical garlic - According to Dr. Sebi, garlic possesses antiviral and alkaline characteristics that are effective against both herpes strains. A fresh garlic clove should be crushed and diluted with olive oil. For up to three days, apply this mixture to the afflicted region.

- Apple cider vinegar (ACV) topically has antiviral and anti-inflammatory effects. Apply a solution of one part ACV to three parts warm water to the afflicted region.

How to follow the Dr. Sebi diet:

- Rule 1. Dr. Sebi's diet should be your main course meal
- Rule 2. Drink a lot of water every day, nothing less than 3.5 litres daily.
- Rule 3. Dr. Sebi's supplements should be taken an hour before any medications.
- Rule 4. No animal products are permitted.
- Rule 5. No alcohol is allowed.
- Rule 6. Abstain from wheat products and only consume the "natural-growing grains" listed in the guide.
- Rule 7. The microwave should not be used to prevent killing the nutrients in your food.
- Rule 8. Abstain from canned or seedless fruits.

BOOK 13
Doctor Sebi's Cure for Herpes PART II

How to Cure Herpes Simplex Virus with Dr. Sebi's Alkaline diet

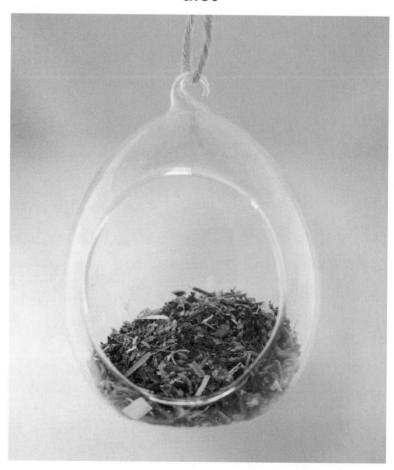

Dr. Sebi's Herpes Cure

Diet changes

Most of the foods we eat nowadays are processed, and some are even canned. While not wholly terrible, many foods already include certain preservatives and chemicals that may not benefit the body. Therefore, eating natural foods like fruits and vegetables is the first step in treating any condition.

These natural meals will assist in removing toxins from your system and have no negative side effects. Your body will be better equipped to fight off the herpes simplex virus if you work to strengthen your immune system by adhering to the suggested diet and avoiding certain substances. Herpes breakouts within your body might be avoided by altering your diet.

Due to the absence of beans, lentils, animal products, and soy products, this particular nutrition guide has a low protein content. You need to purchase Dr. Sebi's cell food supplements in addition to this diet to cleanse and nourish your body and cells.

- Vegetables high in antioxidants - Eat vegetables high in antioxidants to strengthen your immune system and reduce inflammation. Vegetables, including spinach, kale, tomatoes, and cauliflower, are high in antioxidants that bind free radicals and contain more lysine than arginine. This ratio of amino acids aids in herpes suppression.

- Omega-3 fatty acids are abundant in salmon, flaxseed, mackerel, and chia seeds. These fatty acids support your immune system's ability to combat serious inflammatory diseases.

- Consuming foods like oats, almonds, and eggs in healthy amounts balances your body's systems and help your body fight off the herpes virus and other viruses. Saturated fats should not be present in your diet.

- Vitamin C: A adequate intake of vitamin C shortens the period between herpes outbreaks and, over time, helps to heal them.

- Without significantly increasing your lysine intake, brightly colored fruits and vegetables, including bell peppers, oranges, strawberries, papaya, and mango, are particularly high in vitamin C.

- With zinc treatment, you experience fewer herpes outbreaks and have longer intervals between them. Wheat germ and chickpeas are two foods that contain zinc.

B vitamin complex: Foods like broccoli, spinach, and eggs are good sources of B vitamins. These can strengthen your immune system, assisting your body in its battle against the herpes simplex virus.

- L-arginine - Avoid eating foods with high arginine content whenever and however you can. This amino acid, which is highly abundant in chocolate, can aggravate herpes symptoms. If you must, indulge your sweet need with a fruit high in vitamins, such as dried mango or apricots.
- Added sugar: Sugars are converted to acid by your body. Avoid any sugar and meals with added sugar and instead, think about using fruits like bananas and oranges as desserts.

Processed or preservative-rich foods: In general, canned food and other processed foods include artificial preservatives that may increase the risk of oxidative stress. When oxidative damage is kept to a minimum, healing during outbreaks may be more efficient. Stay completely away from these processed foods and frozen meals, and also refrain from grain products and candies in your diet.

- Alcohol - Alcohol degrades the body and raises blood sugar levels. When sugar consumption is excessive, it suppresses white blood cells and significantly lowers the body's ability to fight disease, which increases the likelihood of outbreaks.

Topical Herbs, Oils, and Other Solutions

Some topicals, can help speed up healing, relieve itching, and numb discomfort when used correctly.

- Topical substances that have not been diluted can burn through your skin barrier. These include things like essential oils. Carrier oils like coconut and jojoba ensure the safety of topical medicines.

- Before applying it completely, you should try it on another body part. This precautionary step is designed to prevent you from putting irritating material in a sensitive area of the body.

- Follow the instructions below to do a basic patch test:

- On your forearm, rub the topical.

- Observe for a full day.

- If you experience discomfort, itching, or inflammation, thoroughly cleanse the area and stop using it.

- It is okay to apply to any damaged body parts if you don't notice any symptoms after 24 hours.

- Get a carrier for the topical products listed below: witch hazel, lemon balm extract, neem extract, and essential oils of ginger, tea tree, thyme, eucalyptus, and chamomile.

- Tea tree oil: Genital herpes can be cured with the help of this highly effective antiviral substance. Before applying tea tree oil to the sores to treat HSV, it must first be diluted with carrier oil.

- Wiccan Hazel Importantly, witch hazel has antiviral qualities. While some individuals may use pure witch hazel without irritation, others have an adverse reaction. If your skin is sensitive, you should use a diluted solution.

- **Aloe vera:** Has characteristics that speed the healing of wounds. Furthermore, these qualities can treat herpes lesions. There is no need to dilute pure aloe vera gel; it may be applied straight to any body area.

- **Manuka Honey:** When used topically, manuka honey is virtually as successful in treating HSV-1 and HSV-2 as acyclovir. Manuka honey can be administered straight without the requirement for carrier oil without dilution.

- Herpes simplex can be treated with goat milk since it has antiviral characteristics. Apply directly to the afflicted area.

- Chamomile essential oil: Chamomile essential oil must be diluted with a carrier oil, and some studies indicate that it has calming and virus-fighting characteristics that may help cure HSV-2.

- Ginger essential oil - Ginger essential oil has to be diluted with a carrier oil and can destroy the herpes virus on contact.

- Thyme essential oil - Thyme essential oil should be diluted with a carrier oil and can combat the herpes virus as well.

- Greek sage oil: Diluted with a carrier oil, Greek sage oil aids in treating the herpes virus.

- Eucalyptus oil: Eucalyptus oil has great potential as a herpes treatment. It must be diluted with a carrier oil and has additional healing and soothing properties.

- Carvacrol, a potent antiviral component, is included in Mexican oregano oil, which has to be diluted with carrier oil.

- Lemon balm extract: This oil is essentially used for breakouts and lowers the danger of transmission, but it must first be diluted with carrier oil.

- Sage and rhubarb extract combined—This extract is crucial for treating HSV-1 and should be diluted with a carrier oil before usage.

- Licorice extract: The active component in licorice has antiviral and anti-inflammatory properties. Due to these characteristics, licorice extract works well to cure herpes outbreaks. Direct application is possible without dilution.

- Echinacea extract - Echinacea extract is a very effective antiviral that can combat both herpes simplex strains. It is also an anti-inflammatory, which may help to reduce the severity of current outbreaks. It can be applied straight away.

- **Echinacea extract:** Echinacea extract is a very useful antiviral that can fight against both strains of herpes simplex, and it's also an anti-inflammatory, which may soothe existing outbreaks. It can be used without dilution.

- Neem extract - Pure Neem extract is very viable and may burn your skin if not diluted. You have to cut it with carrier oil.

Tips for Outbreak Management.

To manage a cold sore, follow the steps below:

- Get a new toothbrush and throw away your old one.

- Take plenty of zinc and vitamin C pills, especially if you're under a lot of stress.

- Use a hypoallergenic clear lip balm to shield your skin from the wind, sun, and cold.

- During the epidemic, refrain from sharing cups or beverages.
- While the cold sore is healing, refrain from popping, draining, or otherwise tampering with it.
- How to Control an Outbreak of Genital Herpes.
- Always dress comfortably, using loose-fitting clothes.
- Long, warm showers are a must, and the afflicted region must always be kept dry and clean.
- Avoid taking baths or hot tubs.
- Avoid having sex. Even if you wear a condom, the infection might still spread.

Dr. Sebi's Products and Herbs to Treat Herpes

Dr. Sebi's nutritional guide details specific foods allowed on a diet. These foods are as follows.

- Fruits: Cantaloupe, currants, dates, elderberries, papayas, berries, peaches, pears, plums, key limes, prickly pears, seeded melons, Latin or West Indies, tamarind, and soursop

- Okra, sea vegetables, avocado, bell peppers, cactus flowers, dandelion greens, cucumber, kale, lettuce (excluding iceberg), olives, squash, cherry and plum tomatoes, and zucchini are some examples of vegetables.

- Grains include amaranth, wild rice, rye, spelled, teff, quinoa, and funio.

- Walnuts, Brazil nuts, raw sesame seeds, raw tahini butter, and hemp seeds are some examples of nuts and seeds.

- Among the oils are hemp oil, avocado oil, grapeseed oil, coconut oil (uncooked), sesame oil, and olive oil.

- Elderberry, tila, burdock, ginger, raspberry, chamomile, and fennel are a few herbal teas.

- Spices include oregano, thyme, powdered seaweed, basil, cloves, bay leaf, dill, sweet basil, achiote, cayenne, habanero, tarragon, onion powder, sage, and pure agave syrup. Date sugar also has no added sugar.

- You may also drink a lot of water in addition to tea to speed up your metabolism.

- Grains in pasta, bread, cereal, or flour are OK to eat. Any food leavened with yeast or baking powder is strictly forbidden.

- Foods not on the strict list of permitted foods for the diet outlined below should be avoided.

- Breakfast consists of two banana-spelled pancakes with agave syrup.

- Snack: 1 cup of a green juice smoothie made with kale, apples, cucumbers, and ginger.
- Lunch will consist of a kale salad with tomatoes, onions, avocado, dandelion greens, chickpeas, basil dressing, and olive oil.
- Fruit and herbal tea for a snack.
- Dinner will be stir-fried veggies and wild rice.
-

Day 2

- Breakfast consists of a smoothie shake made with water, strawberries, bananas, and hemp seeds.
- Snack: Blueberry muffins made with spelled flour, pure coconut milk, agave syrup, sea salt, and blueberries.
- Pizza made at home with a spelled-flour crust, Brazil-nut cheese, and veggies for lunch
- Snack: Sliced red peppers on the side and rye toast with tahini butter.
- Dinner will be a flatbread made of spelled wheat with a chickpea burger, onions, tomatoes, and kale.
-

Day 3

For breakfast, cook quinoa with peaches, agave syrup, and pure coconut milk.

Tea with chamomile, grapes with seeds, and sesame seeds.

Lunch: a salad spelled with diced veggies, olive oil, and key lime dressing.

Snack: A banana, mango, and pure coconut milk smoothie.

Dinner will be a fresh vegetable soup with water, kale, onions, red peppers, mushrooms, zucchini, and powdered seaweed.

Why Dr. Sebi's Cure for Herpes is the Best Option?

The Dr. Sebi diet encourages consuming entire, unprocessed, and plant-based meals, which boosts the body's natural immunity.

Given that every medicine is entirely natural, it could help with weight reduction and has no negative side effects.

In addition, Dr. Sebi's diet advises people to consume real foods rather than processed ones to boost their immunity and improve their body's nutritional worth. It is also advantageous, particularly when you adhere to it rigorously, since it encourages you to adopt a healthy eating pattern that is more plant-based and affects the microbiome or the collection of intestinal bacteria. The body has a lower risk of getting sick when fewer germs are present.

The Dr. Sebi diet aids with appetite management. A study was done, and it was shown that eating a plant-based diet makes you feel more energized, active, and pleased.

The greatest herpes treatment is Dr. Sebi's since it not only treats herpes simplex but also controls and strengthens defenses against other disease-causing bacteria and maintains a stable pH level in your body. Your complete body remains healthy with Dr. Sebi's treatment and nutrition.

BOOK 14
How to Stop Smoking
Made Simple

Without Gaining Weight Using Dr Sebi's Alkaline Diet

Preface

You hold a book in your hands that organically provides tried-and-true methods for curing the smoking sickness. If you have tried several expensive medications and other ways without much success, you still have smoking urges and withdrawal symptoms. Continue reading because the author of this book was a biochemist who was also a naturalist, pathologist, and herbalist before he passed away. He developed this strategy utilizing the alkaline diet after doing an in-depth study on herbs to treat all ailments. Dr. Sebi has long believed that bodily mucus, including smoking, is the root cause of all diseases. This book will aid in your recovery from the sickness of smoking.

A New Way To Stop Smoking

As opposed to the typical way of quitting smoking, where you first feel like you can conquer Mount Everest and then spend the following weeks craving cigarettes or even feeling envious of smokers, you'll feel delighted and ready to take on the world after being healed of a horrific illness. You will reach a point in your life where you even feel in awe of yourself for lighting up. Empathy for those still trying to quit would be all that was left, not envy. This chapter aims to do that. To instill in you the belief that quitting is much simpler than most people realize.

To avoid appearing paradoxical, if you smoke, maintain doing so until you have finished reading this book. Then, you will realize that smoking has no positive effects on your health, which is why. In actuality, the absence of a cigarette makes a smoker want one much more. When permitted, the smoker ponders why they smoke and its impact on them each time they light up. Smokers often struggle with this. So, let's assume you became addicted and think you're addicted whether you want it or not; the only time you can focus or unwind is when you're smoking a cigarette. Since your need for a cigarette will diminish as you read, I kindly ask that you refrain from trying to put an end to it all at once because doing so might be fatal. If you adhere to the advice in this chapter, smoking will soon become a thing for you.

1. Decide that you won't smoke again and keep that commitment.
2. Instead of feeling down about your choice, embrace it.

Smoking is a cunning and evil trap. One may effectively stop smoking by comprehending the myths, delusions, and indoctrination that went along with it; nicotine addiction is not the issue. Only when you are aware of your adversary's strategy can you triumph.

Ex-smokers often say they had weeks of despair when they tried to quit smoking. When they were determined to quit, it got easier over time—say, let's from a hundred a day to none—and they succeeded in doing so without stumbling. Even the detox period grew delightful to the point that they no longer had a yearning for cigarettes. They seem to have a fresh lease on life. Their lives now make more sense, and they are happier than ever.

You won't realize you'll likely continue smoking for the rest of your life if you don't stop smoking until you've given your smoking problem some serious thought. You won't be able to view smoking for what it is until you come to this awareness. It contributes nothing to your life and is dirty.

Few ex-smokers would admit to having those strange cravings for a cigarette, but it's not important enough to worry about. Others, on the other hand, might claim that they don't miss smoking because they are currently enjoying their greatest life. They can handle the pressure and stress of daily life. As a result, they are unwilling to give up their newfound independence and now attend more social events than ever before.

It is simple to stop smoking without fear of withdrawal symptoms, which is a lovely reality. However, uncertainty and doubts trigger the need to smoke, and hesitation and depression make quitting difficult. Nicotine addicts who smoke can go for a long time leading regular lives without being affected by it. Only when you desire and can have a smoke do you get disturbed and suffer.

Making it simply requires making halting certain and decisive. Be certain right away. Hope and wishing won't cut it. Rejoicing your decision, quit smoking, and keep it up. Before you begin, take these crucial considerations into account.

1. You can do it: You must understand that you are your boss and that no one else has the power to force you to light up the next cigarette.
2. You have nothing to lose and everything to gain, including improved health, more money saved, and attractiveness as opposed to misery. Think about these advantages.
3. The sooner you realize that smoking is a drug addiction, the better. Nothing compares to smoking one cigarette. When you are grumbling about that one cigarette, all you will do is punish yourself needlessly.
4. As I mentioned before, consider smoking a drug addiction that must be treated right now. Not a social custom that might only harm you. You have the illness, and as with any illness, we don't just wish it away; instead, we take action immediately to prevent it from worsening.
5. There must be a distinction between this physiological addiction and the mindset associated with smoking or quitting smoking. All smokers would seize the chance to return to the moment they first became addicted. You are no longer a smoker once you decide this will be your final cigarette. Don't hold out for any unique emotions. Without feeling down about your choice, go out and enjoy life. You are no longer that miserable smoker that is ruining their life. You are the one who suddenly appreciates life's beauty and is hesitant to give it up.

After making the ultimate choice to stop smoking, the three weeks of withdrawal would be much easier if you were in the appropriate state of mind.

If, after going over those mentioned above, you still feel doomed, the following may be the cause:

1. You worry that you won't succeed. Avoid worrying about this phobia. Just keep reading to find out how much smoking might be used as a confidence trick.
   Only a fool already aware of the ploy continues to delude himself. The sensible ones, however, simply fail to fall for the confidence ploy. As long as you can overcome your fear of failing, you will succeed.
2. Perhaps the information discussed did not yet make sense to you. Eliminate any doubts you may have. Do well to review the five criteria mentioned above.
3. even though you wholeheartedly concur with the topic, you continue to feel terrible. This is a warning sign that something bad is about to happen. So, smile since you've already gained some ground.

So, set yourself up for success by seeing yourself as a non-smoker and maintaining that identity.

Dr Sebi's Approach to Quit Smoking

Herbal supplements are one method of quitting smoking; they are administered to lessen cravings and withdrawal from nicotine. In addition, the tissues that smoking has harmed can be repaired with these therapies.

The most popular herbal treatment for desire management, among other things, is green tea, which may be consumed all day long. Green tea assists in keeping the body stocked with substances that lessen the desire to smoke during detoxification. Green tea and Lobelia tea can be consumed during the detoxifying process. However, it is advisable to speak with a doctor before using this herbal supplement since, if taken improperly, it may damage your health.

Important minerals, including vitamin C, vitamin D, and calcium, are blocked by smoking. One cigarette, for instance, depletes the body of 25 milligrams of vitamin C. Adding more fruits and vegetables to your diet can help you replenish these nutrients. Some studies have revealed that it may also help you stop desiring cigarettes. In addition, food starts to taste better, and the flavors are more discernible once you stop smoking.

According to some studies, ginseng may help treat nicotine addiction because it may lessen the effects of dopamine, a neurotransmitter linked to pleasure in the brain that is released when a person smokes. As a result, ginseng tea may lessen the desire to smoke and make smoking less pleasurable.

Smokers have claimed that drinking milk made cigarettes taste even worse; most smokers acknowledged that it left their smoke with a harsh flavor. Consuming milk and other dairy products might make cigarettes taste unpleasant while experiencing a need, which may help you quit smoking.

Since quitting smoking is linked to weight gain, you need carefully pay attention to your nutrition. Otherwise, you can discover that you're substituting healthy food for smoke, which keeps your hands and mouth occupied. You may also be used to the appetite-suppressing and metabolism-boosting effects of nicotine, which cause people to weigh somewhat less when they smoke than when they stop.

Consider including high fiber beans in your diet if you find gaining weight frustrating. Additionally, honey is crucial in the process of quitting smoking. It is bursting with healthy proteins, enzymes, and vitamins.

The Importance Of Detox And Revitalizing Your Body

Congratulations on your choice to stop smoking, first and foremost. The challenge's most challenging section has just been overcome. The additional toxins accumulated over time must subsequently be removed from the body. The Dr. Sebi alkaline diet and recipes are jam-packed with these substances. Herbal detox is the best technique to eliminate these harmful toxins from your body.

Effects of cigarette chemicals on the human body

Every time you smoked, hundreds of pollutants were breathed into your body. Approximately 4,000 chemical agents and 60 carcinogens were inhaled into your lungs and spread throughout your entire body via the bloodstream. The most prevalent of these poisons, nicotine, is the main factor in the emergence of lung cancer. In addition, smoking may cause several ailments, including chronic bronchitis, bladder cancer, stomach cancer, cervical cancer, and stroke. You are also at risk of getting these conditions.

So, what is Detox and why it is important?

Detoxifying involves removing extra toxins and additives that might hurt the body. This goes beyond limiting your food, which most individuals do for a brief time before reverting to their previous bad behaviors. Simply said, detoxing is a fresh start. It is a method for purging negative emotions and mental patterns from our minds. Removing heavy metals from the body through detoxification also helps to enhance brain clarity, digestion, and general health.

Since we frequently come into contact with toxins in our daily lives, detoxing is also an opportunity to eliminate harmful substances, including toxic attitudes, behaviors, and emotions.

Detoxing also allows us to pause, reflect, and review every aspect of our lives, including our routines, eating habits, personal cleanliness, and everything in between.

Benefits of Detoxing After you stop smoking

The following are also some of the benefits enjoyed by an ex-smoker:

- ➢ Increased energy

- ➢ Metabolism-boosting usually associated with quitting

- ➢ Improved respiration

- ➢ Weight loss

- ➢ Looking younger, feeling younger

How to Detox your body?

You need to use herbal detox to clear up your body's major organs to be safe now that you've quit smoking. The goal is to stop pollutants accumulated over time from festering and endangering your health. If pollutants are not eliminated, your health may suffer. Toxins likely to be released through the skin, bowel movements, and urine will be flushed out by eliminating these dangerous compounds using herbs and other natural procedures. Additionally, eating fruits and veggies whole does wonder for detoxifying your body.

Food You Should and Should Not Eat To Detox Your Body

Food to Eat

These meals aid in reducing the urge to smoke. By changing the flavor of smoking, they only make it appear awful. Natural foods should be consumed for detoxifying, such as

The greatest things to eat when detoxifying your body are fruits, vegetables, beans, seeds, whole grains, and nuts. Vegetables and fruits include elements that act as powerful detoxification agents and digestive enzymes. Because they are high in fiber, whole grains, vegetables, fruits, and beans aid in removing toxins from the body through the colon. Due to their abundance of fat-soluble vitamins, nuts and seeds assist in stimulating brain cells. Additionally, nuts and seeds enhance the way that brain cells work in general. All of these foods are abundant in antioxidants, vitamins, and minerals, enabling the body to flush out toxins. This nutrient-rich meal can make the body feel better overall by being consumed.

Lemons, rich in vitamin C, are the fruit of choice for individuals trying to detox. These antioxidant works wonder to combat free radicals. The body may suffer as a result of this. Lemons have an alkaline impact that aids in re-establishing the body's PH balance, enhancing the immune system. Starting your detox with a simple lemon slice in hot water is an excellent idea.

Ginger is another excellent detox meal since it helps digestion and lessens bloating and gas. In addition, it has a lot of antioxidants, which help to strengthen your immune system.

Despite its strong odor, garlic is excellent for detoxifying the body. It has antiviral, antibacterial, and antibiotic effects, as well as allicin, which promotes the creation of white blood cells, a defense mechanism for the body against infections. It is best eaten uncooked. It assists your liver in producing enzymes designed to remove toxins from your body when mixed with onions.

Artichokes are another fantastic meal. They include plenty of fiber and antioxidants. In addition, they promote liver function and aid in the digestion of fatty meals.

The best meals for a perfect detox are said to include watercress. It includes detoxifying minerals, including vitamins, zinc, potassium, and antioxidants. Additionally, diuretic in nature, watercress aids in the removal of pollutants. Watercress can assist smokers in getting rid of cancer-causing substances from their bodies.

Active components can be found in green tea. This aids in detoxification and offers extra health advantages. For example, antioxidants included in green tea assist the body get rid of pollutants. Green tea also improves liver function and helps shield the liver from illness.

Cabbage is another excellent detox meal. Sulforaphane, a substance found in cabbage, helps the body fight against pollutants. Additionally, glutathione, an antioxidant that supports liver health, is present in cabbage.

Cucumber, which contains 90% water, is a fantastic way to enhance your body's water content. It also aids with digestion.

Supplements: Several supplements available can assist smokers in getting through the detoxification and withdrawal stages. The clearance of nicotine is accelerated by acidic urine, which raises the want for more. A diet high in alkaline also slows down nicotine detoxification while reducing the desire to smoke.

Multivitamins: We first require vitamin B, which is typically deficient in smokers. mostly B1, B6, and B12. B3 aids in releasing nicotine-constricted blood vessels. By lowering the body's cholesterol levels, vitamin B3 also helps lower the chance of developing atherosclerosis. B12, in contrast, works to lessen the cellular harm nicotine and tars produce.

Pantothenic acid aids in slowing down skin aging. Additionally crucial are folic acid, chlorine, and coenzyme Q10.

Zinc, magnesium, molybdenum, and copper are additional vital minerals needed throughout the detoxification process.

Food Not To Eat

It is in your best interest to be aware that some meals might cause cravings for tobacco and function as a trigger. If you must eat certain items, it is also crucial for you to make a strategy in advance to control your urges. The worst foods for a detox diet include

those containing caffeine, meat, dairy, alcohol, and wheat. Alcohol damages the liver and lowers the amounts of minerals that aid in detoxification, such as zinc and magnesium.

Your gut microbes are bred by meat. Both digestion and bowel movement are slowed down by it. Wheat is harmful to the intestinal lining. This results in inadequate nutritional intake. Consuming gluten promotes intestinal irritation, which results in bloating, gas, and constipation.

Poor cell function is caused by dairy products like milk, cheese, and cheese. They impede detoxification because they are acidic to the body, whereas caffeine causes the body's toxic levels to rise.

Additionally, processed, packaged, and frozen meals should be avoided during detoxing since they are heavy in salt, sugar, unhealthy fats, and artificial chemicals.

High salt intake harms blood pressure. Both the detoxification process and cell activity are slowed down by it. Dietary sugar worsens brain fog and energy peaks and valleys and makes mood swings more common. Additionally, sugar competes against healthy microorganisms in the gut, which slows down detoxification. Many artificial components are manufactured from petrochemicals, while unhealthy fats stress the liver and your waistline. They are difficult to digest and metabolize and toxic to the liver.

Dr. Sebi's Stop Smoking Diet Recipes

One must reduce their smoking habits if one wishes to lead a healthy lifestyle. The examples that follow from Dr. Sebi's smoking diet formula assist in putting it into practice.

1. Lemon and dried ginger

Ginger's sulfur-containing component aids in reducing smoking addiction. A little piece of ginger should be soaked in lemon juice. After that, add black pepper to it, and combine before storing. Suck on the piece of ginger whenever you feel the need or craving to smoke, and you will be OK.

2. Onion juice

Any smoker who has made several attempts to stop smoking but has been unsuccessful might benefit from drinking onion juice three times per day to help control their urges.

3. Ginseng

Ginseng does more than only reduce the desire to smoke. It also aids in easing withdrawal symptoms. Stress on the body and mind might manifest as this symptom.

4. Beeswax and dalchini

Because both honey and dalchini offer health benefits that can aid in quitting smoking, taking some dalchini powder combined with half a teaspoon of honey with water will help reduce the desire to smoke.

5. Harad/Harar

The black harad, which shrinks in size after a brief soaking in water, can reduce the desire to smoke. Simply take it and put it in your mouth for a few minutes whenever hunger strikes, and you will be fine.

6. Drink some milk.

Studies at Duke University have shown that drinking milk before smoking makes the smokes taste worse. Therefore, if the temptation for cigarettes strikes, drink some milk or consume any dairy item, such as yogurt. You won't smoke for a very long time, thanks to this.

Others include

Grapefruit is beneficial to the skin. It provides effective pore cleansing, which is crucial after quitting smoking. Grapefruit is a powerful antioxidant that helps to prevent cancer, lower blood acidity, and heal damage to the lungs. It is nutrient-rich and aids in reducing the negative effects of free radicals. It safeguards the lungs, reduces the danger of heart disease, and helps maintain oral health.

Ginger is a plant that helps the body cleanse. Strong antioxidants like those found in ginger aid in the fight against cancer. Ginger aids in removing the harmful chemicals in tobacco after you stop smoking. Ginger is excellent for digestion and prevents heartburn, bloating, and stomach reflux. In addition to providing energy, ginger also aids in the body's detoxification of cigarette poisons.

It also relieves anxiety and increases sweat due to ginger's warming properties. This removes the poisons from the body and reduces the number of dangerous compounds in the blood. Furthermore, it aids in the treatment of smoking withdrawal symptoms, such as nausea. Additionally, Dr. Sebi's turmeric ginger mixture might aid in quitting smoking. Finally, it aids in the body's detoxification from all the damaging toxins that might result in several diseases.

Green vegetables are abundant in magnesium, a mineral in which smokers are deficient—these leafy greens aid in clearing the body of tobacco's damaging effects. In addition, green veggies provide you with fresh air and aid in skin recovery.

ACE: This beverage is anti-smoking. Ace is derived from the combination of the vitamins A, C, and E in oranges, carrots, and lemons. The carrot aids in preventing skin aging and promotes skin healing. Oranges are potent antioxidants with vitamins and minerals that help prevent winter illnesses.

Another diet plan using the valerian root has potent sedative qualities. These characteristics make it easier to manage nicotine withdrawal symptoms. Symptoms of stress, worry, and agitation. Natural cure valerian is particularly good at reducing cravings for nicotine.

Cayenne pepper: In addition to being a rich source of antioxidants, it aids in desensitising the respiratory system to all addictive substances. This stabilises the lung membrane while simultaneously repairing damaged lungs. Cayenne pepper reduces the desire to smoke cigarettes.

Is Dr. Sebi's Stop Smoking Diet Effective?

When successfully quitting smoking, Dr. Sebi's diet has a track record of success and is widely regarded. Dr. Sebi's stop smoking diet is the most successful assistance program available for smokers. This is a plant-based, alkaline diet that can restore lost nutrients and heal organs that have been harmed by smoking. The abundance of antioxidant compounds in its fruits, veggies, and whole-grain meals will help you get back to good health. In addition, the diet's vitamins A, C, and E, beta-carotene, and selenium can help lower the risk of cancer and other smoking-related disorders.

Dr. Sebi's stop-smoking diet includes water as a key component. It balances out the dehydrating effects of smoking. Depending on the water content of the veggies, salad, and fruits eaten, a 2 to 3-quart intake is needed. In addition, the mildly acidic state in the body brought on by smoking can be balanced with an alkaline quit-smoking diet.

This fiber-rich alkaline diet for quitting smoking aids in detoxification. This is achieved through sustaining bowel movements, which are necessary for the body to flush dangerous substances out.

During the detoxification and withdrawal, Dr. Sebi's alkaline diet for quitting smoking was successful. By increasing blood alkalinity, made possible by consuming raw food, fruits, and vegetables, raw food intake lowers cravings and interest in smoking. An alkaline stop-smoking diet is a huge booster during the withdrawal stage, contrary to what is also supported by several research. This diet does not need to be followed for the rest of one's life.

Last, Dr. Sebi's stop-smoking diet is quick, long-lasting, and successful for heavy smokers. No need to be concerned about gaining any weight. Additionally, it delays the removal of nicotine from the body, which lessens the urge to smoke and aids in controlling cravings.

Why Dr. Sebi's Stop Smoking Diet is the Best Option

Medical professionals from Columbia University in the USA conducted a study. The most frequent smokers have the highest acid balance in their bodies, according to research on the amount of acidity or alkalinity in a smoker's body. Because their bodies are more acidic, nicotine exits the body more quickly, which explains why they need another cigarette more quickly after the last one. However, because an alkaline diet lowers the pace at which the nicotine content exits the body, it makes it simpler to stop smoking by reducing cigarette cravings.

The alkaline diet was tested on a group of smokers at the University of Nebraska Medical Center in the USA for five weeks. At the end of the trial, all except one had given up smoking; the remaining person was only smoking two cigarettes per day.

According to the investigation results mentioned above, the alkaline diet (also known as Dr. Sebi's alkaline diet) is the most effective method for quitting smoking.

BOOK 15
DR. SEBI Anxiety
Remedies

Intro Duction to Dr. Sebi's anxiety remedies

Anxiety and stress can cause a variety of health problems and mental illnesses. It is essential to address anxiety when it occurs in order to prevent escalation, detriment, and long-term impact. While modern medicine is focused on clinical diagnosis and pharmaceutical intervention, there are many easy ways to avoid the dangers of anxiety and treatment, as well as benefit from related favorable health benefits. It is natural to feel anxious, worried, or fearful in some situations. These feelings are our bodies' natural 'fight or flight response' to a perceived dangerous or perilous circumstance. However, if persistent feelings of anxiety interfere with your capacity to live a normal life, you may have an anxiety disorder.

Anxiety is your body's reaction to anticipated danger. It is frequently associated with worry or fear and is accompanied by cognitive issues such as difficulties concentrating and physical symptoms such as nausea, hakng, and mild tenseness. Anxiety can be a normal reaction to some events, but some anxiety is part of an anxiety disorder.

There are several types of anxiety disorders, and they all have similar symptoms, with some differences. It may feel as if your anxiety symptoms are controlling your life, whether that means fear of a panic attack, avoiding people due to social anxiety, or simply a constant feeling of concern and agitation. Understanding the symptoms of your unique type of anxiety will assist you in seeking the best appropriate treatment and improving your quality of life.

The Best Tips From Dr. Sebi's Methodology

1. Eat Close To Nature: Like your ancestors did. Eating should not be a chore, and we all tend to overcomplicate things. So, let's strip it down to the bac. Before modern medicine poked its nose into our food and, consequently, our health, our forefathers knew what was good for them. Stick to the foods recommended by Dr. Sebi's Nutritional Guide and you'll be fine.

2. Be Consistent: Consistency is key. Unfortunately, one week of eating like a healthy god/goddess will not result in three weeks of eating like a kid in a candy hoop. Dr. Sebi did not believe in eating "bad things" (ugar, hybrids, animal products, alcohol, coffee, etc.) in moderation, becaue even the smallest amount of thoe ubtance may me up the alkalne environment that t'optmal for healing, so you should stick to what Dr. Sebi has suggested.

3. Drink More Water: The odds are, you're not drinking enough water. Dr. Sebi has recommended drinking one gallon of purified water every day, so get started!

4. Detox And Replenish: After years of poor eating habits, the cells in your body have accumulated toxins, which cause inflammation, mucous, weariness, and, finally, potentially fatal disease. The Afrcan Bo-mneral Balance n Dr. Seb' Cell Food product will detox each cells and replace depleted minerals, allowing rebuilding and rejuvenation to take place.

5. Avoid Raw Sugar: According to Dr. Sebi, raw sugar is one of the worst things you can ingest in your body, therefore avoid it completely. Date sugar and agave syrup in small amounts are permitted.

Explanation Of Anxiety

Anxiety is a sensation of unease, worry, or fear that, when persistent and affecting daily life, may be an indication of an anxiety disorder. Anxiety can be a debilitating condition that affects every aspect of your life, from how you think about yourself to your relationships and physical changes. Know that there is assistance available for anxiety. Anxiety is treatable, and many people may work through their anxiety symptoms with a specific treatment plan that may include medication, therapy, lifestyle changes, and healthy eating habits.

What Is Anxiety?

The "Diagnostic and Statistical Manual of Mental Disorders" (DSM-5) defines anxiety as the expectation of a future threat. Everyone feels anxious at some time in their lives, but not everyone suffers from an anxiety condition. There are several types of anxiety disorders, including generalized anxiety, social anxiety, and others. These conditions should not be exacerbated by day-to-day anxiety. Anxiety is our bodies' natural response to stress, and most people will experience it on occasion.

However, it may become a problem when it begins to interfere with your day-to-day existence. Read on to find out how you can assist and minimize anxiety. Anxiety is a complicated ailment that most people find difficult to explain. It's not something that can be readily defined in a dictionary, and individuals who have never experienced anxiety may not grasp what it means to have it.

It's natural to be nervous about important events, such as a job interview, a performance evaluation, a first date, a huge exam, delivery, or any number of other life events. Worrying, on the other hand, may sometimes spiral out of control and become an anxiety disorder. Anxiety disorders are diagnosable mental health conditions characterized by excessive fear, anxiety, and accompanying behavioral and physical changes that may occur over time. These conditions have a physical and mental influence on daily activities such as school, employment, leisure, and relationships.

Causes Of Anxiety

Anxiety is caused by more than one thing; it can impact people in a variety of ways. Many different variables can contribute to the development of mental health disorders such as anxiety disorder. These factor nclude biological factor (for each genetc, the experence of chronc phycal llne or damage and pychologcal or ocal factor (experiences of tranc They can include, but are not limited to:

1. Past Or Childhood Experiences

It's typical for things that happened in the past to cause worry in a child, adolescent, or adult during the moment, as well as for many years afterwards. These experiences include physical or emotional abuse, neglect, being bullied or socially outcast, or losing a parent.

2. Current Life Situations

Anxiety can be caused by current life events or concerns. Some examples include having to work long hours, feeling lonely, having money issues, being unemployed, feeling the strain of studying, or feeling weary.

3. New And Existing Physical Or Mental Health Problems

These might make people feel worried or aggravate their anxiety. Anxiety might be caused by an ongoing health issue, Serou. It's also common for people to acquire anxiety when coping with mental health issues, such as depression.

4. Drugs Or Medication

Anxiety can be a consequence of some mental or physical health medicines, recreational drugs, or alcohol.

Psychological Explanations of Anxiety Disorders

Merely having a biological predisposition or heightened sensitivity to stress is insufficient to develop an anxiety disorder. As previously stated, a person is more likely to develop an anxiety disorder if they are biologically predisposed to anxiety in conjunction with a psychological sensitivity. Research has identified four major psychological variables that predispose people to anxiety. These are:

- Cognitive Distortions

- Cognitive Appraisals

- Cognitive Beliefs

- Perceived Control

Risk Factors Of Anxiety

Risks-factors-of-anxiety even though anyone can experience anxiety at any given moment, there are a few risk factors of anxiety to look out for. Some of these risk factors of anxiety include:

- Personality: Certain personalities, such as introversion, are more prone to developing anxiety disorder.

- Substance abuse: Withdrawal from ubtance or ongoing alcohol and drug abuse might result in anxiety problems.

- Being Female: Statistics show that anxiety disorders are more frequent among women.

- Trauma: Childhood or even adult trauma can result in anxiety disorder.

- Stre: Whether it is stress from a pre-existing disease or stress from regular life, stress is a major risk factor for anxiety.

- Pre-existing mental health disorders, such as depression, are among the leading risk factors for anxiety.

- Family Member: People who have family members who suffer from anxiety disorder are at a higher risk of having it themselves.

- Panic Disorder: A type of persistent anxiety that can lead to an anxiety attack.

- Generalized Anxiety Disorder: Constant anxiety over daily life occurrences.

- Subtance-Induced Anxiety: Anxiety caused by alcohol or drugs.

- Agoraphoba: Anxiety about locations on vtng place, followed by loss of control and thoughts of being imprisoned.

- Separation Anxiety Disorder: Commonly found in children, it causes anxiety due to the fear of long parental or parental figure.

Signs and Symptoms Of Anxiety

Anxiety can impact how you feel physically or mentally, as well as cause behavioral changes. It might be difficult to recognise when worry is interfering with how you feel or act. Anxiety frequently causes a mix of physical, psychological, and social symptoms. Your precise profile will differ depending on your situation, kind of anxiety disorder, and personal triggers. Now that we know what the definitions of anxiety are, as well as the risk factor for anxiety, let's look at the signs and ymptom of anxiety. Keep a look out for the following signs and symptoms:

Physical Symptoms Of Anxiety

- Sweating and hot flushes
- Increased or irregular heartbeat
- Faster breathing that is hard to control
- Headaches and other aches throughout the body
- Nausea and loss of appetite

Mental Symptoms Of Anxiety

- Feeling emotional
- Increased anxiety about the past and future, but also the inability to stop worrying about everything (e.g., fear that people can see you are nervous, people are angry with you, the danger of a panic attack).
- Feeling tense, nervous, and unable to relax
- Insomnia
- Ruminating on bad experiences

Behavioral Changes Caused By Anxiety

- Problems with your concentration that may be affecting your work
- Inability to form or maintain relationships

- Not taking care of yourself

- Worries about trying new things

- Feeling you can't nj any leisure or downtime

The Dangers of Anxiety And Stress

What are the harms of suffering from chronic stress and anxiety? Let's find out!

- Ulcers

- Panic attacks

- Chronic fatigue

- Respiratory disorders

- Heart disease

- Irritable Bowel Syndrome

- Chronic diseases

- Chronic obstructive pulmonary disease

- Migraines

5 Simple Tips To Avoid Many Risks Associated With Anxiety And Stress

Because the long-term impact of anxiety can be severe, it is critical to treat anxiety early and frequently in order to avoid and reduce the risk of catastrophic side effects. Follow these 5 easy steps to prevent the hazards of anxiety and stress:

1. Make Time For Yourself: Modern life is expensive, and sometimes we just need to slow down and relax. Taking time to relax and detach from the world is essential for managing chronic stress and anxiety. At the end of the day, relax and enjoy your favorite activity, such as spending time with loved ones or drinking a cup of Dr. Seb' Stre Relief Herbal Tea.

2. Make Time For What Makes You Happy: Life does not have to be all work and no play! Make time for what you enjoy. Try to do something every day that makes you feel good, and it will help you recover from your trauma. It doesn't have to be a long time; perhaps 15 to 20 minutes would suffice.

3. Workout: Working exercise on a daily basis is one of the finest ways to calm your body and mind. It doesn't have to be strenuous exercise, but going for a stroll after dinner or stretching before bed can significantly boost your mood.

4. Eat Healthily: Stress may have an impact on your body's natural defenses, but eating the correct foods can help. It's natural to feel drained at times by the stress of daily life, and unfortunately, we tend to go for junk food, but high-calorie or calorie-dense foods just deceive us into thinking we feel better. Eating good foods and exercising regularly can provide significant stress alleviation.

5. DEEP BREATHING: Breathing is such a natural bodily function that most people take it for granted. However, tre may cause people to get into a detrimental cycle of breathing and anxiety. Anxious folks are taking hort, shallow breaths with increasing frequency. While this is a symptom of anxiety, it is also a cause and exacerbates the sense of anxiety. Anxiety causes shallow breathing, which causes more anxiety, which causes shallow breathing, and so on.

As you might imagine, everyone agrees that it is essential to develop healthy breathing habits, and here are some of the primary health benefits of deep breathing that have been discovered:

- Improves core muscle stability
- Lowers your heart rate
- Improves intense exercise capabilities
- Regulates blood pressure
- Lowers harmful effects of cortisol
- Reduces lactic acid build-up
- Increases the volume of oxygen received by the body
- Results in more organized electric patterns in the brain
- Improves energy metabolism
- Allows improved healing capabilities
- Boosts the immune system
- Positively impacts memory
- Calming impact on the brain

Whatever you do, remember that controlling chronic pain and anxiety is as important for good health as any other step you take!

Ways Of Dealing With Anxiety

Finding the correct support and control systems might aid in coping with the problem. The following steps may assist you in managing your anxiety:

1. Talking to someone you trust can help relieve your anxieties, and a listening ear from someone who cares about you can be comforting. If you are unable to chat with someone close, there are free helplines available.

2. Managing your worries might be difficult and, at times, unmanageable. Writing down your fears and storing them away will help you get rid of them for a while. If you're anxious about negative things happening, set out a specific time to reassure yourself that you've thought about them at least once that day.

3. Taking care of oneself via adequate rest, nutritious food, and regular exercise has been shown to have a positive impact on both physical and mental well-being.

4. Breathing Exercises: Letting your breath flow deep into your belly can also help you control your anxiety. Count to five as you breathe in through your nose and out through your mouth. Rep this for up to five minutes.

5. Keeping a diary allows you to track how you feel when you are anxious, and you may pick up on what triggers the feeling.

6. Seeking help from others who have gone through or are going through something similar allows you to learn from others. It also serves as a helpful reminder that you are not the only one going through what you are going through.

7. Using complementary and alternative therapies can also be quite beneficial for certain people. Yoga, massage, and herbal therapy, for example, are just a few of the therapy's individuals use to help them relax and sleep better. There are also alternative therapies, such as meditation and hypnotherapy, that can help people relax and let go of their worries. Anxiety might also be beneficial.

8. Regular exercise can also have a positive influence on anxiety levels. Some people find that activities such as swimming, walking, jogging, and yoga help them turn off and relax.

9. Tuning into well-being advice is also a useful method of learning and reminding yourself of some of the things you can do to help with anxiety control, sleep issues, confidence boosting, and more.

10. Listening to relaxation and mental health apps might help if you're looking to learn new things ue and copng tactics or renforce certain things you already know and have

learnt. There are several apps available for you to pick from, ranging from Be Mindful and Beat Panic to Sleep and Feeling Good: Positive Mindset.

Types Of Anxiety Disorders

1. Panic disorder

2. Generalized anxiety disorder

3. Obsessive-compulsive disorder

4. Social anxiety disorder

5. Generalized Anxiety Disorder

6. Other anxiety disorders

7. Post-traumatic stress disorder (PTSD)

People with generalized anxiety disorder (GAD) have excessive and persistent worry, fear, and anxiety that is difficult to control and is detrimental to their well-being. GAD can be diagnosed when these symptoms occur for a significant number of days in a row for at least 6 months.

Symptoms Of GAD Include:

1. Fatigue

2. Irritability

3. Restlessness

4. Difficulty sleeping

5. Muscle tension, soreness, and ache

6. Concentration difficulties

2. Special Anxiety Disorder

Special anxiety disorder, formerly known as social phobia, is characterized by an overwhelming dread of social and performance situations. It's more than just timidity. People who suffer from social anxiety experience tremendous anxiety, which can lead to avoidant behavior while meeting new people, maintaining relationships, speaking in front of others, dining in public, and other activities.

Symptoms Of A Social Anxiety Disorder Include:

- Self-judgment and self-consciousness

- Avoiding social situations or feeling acute fear during them

- Nausea

- Sweating

- Trembling

- Rapid heart rate

- The feeling of "mind going blank"

- Provoke dread and anxiety in one or more social situations.

- Blushing

In youngsters, social anxiety disorder can manifest differently. Obviously, anxiety must occur in peer circumstances for children, not simply with adults. Tantrums, freezng, weeping, clngng, and refusal to speak are all symptoms.

3. Obsessive-Compulsive Disorder

Obsessive-compulsive disorder (OCD) involves repeated, unwanted thoughts that lead to specific and repeatable actions that interfere with daily living. OCD is no longer classified as an anxiety disorder in DSM-5, but it does produce anxiety.

Symptoms Of The Obsessive-Compulsive Disorder Include:

1. Obsession: Thoughts and anxieties that are recognised as excessive yet will not go away. Fear of germ, fear of long omethng, aggreve or taboo thought, yearning for symmetry or order, and other symptoms are common.

2. Compulon: Repetitive behavior undertaken to reduce anxiety and usually tied to obsessions. Counting, exceve cleaning or hand washing, overly prece orderng and arrangng, repeated checking, and more are examples of compulon.

3. Spend at least one hour every day on obesity and compulsion, and they cause severe distress or impairment in essential aspects of your life.

4. Panic Disorder

Panic disorder is a mental health condition characterized by rutorrent and unexpected pac attack. A panic attack is a state of extreme fear and anxiety accompanied by a variety of physical symptoms, which some people describe as feeling like a heart attack.

Symptoms Of A Panic Attack Include:

- Heart palpitations and rapid heart rate

- Feelings of impending doom or death

- Trembling

- Shortness of breath

- Sweating

- Chest pain

- Chills

- Feeling smothered or choked

Panic episodes do not constitute a mental health disorder in and of itself. They occur in a variety of mental health conditions, including Parkinson's disease. Someone with panic disorder will have recurring panic attacks, ongoing fear about future panic attacks, and avoidant behaviors around situations that might trigger a panic attack. To be diagnosed with panic disorder, at least one panic attack must be followed by a month-long period of persistent worry about subsequent attacks or avoidance behaviors.

5. Post-Traumatic Stress Disorder

PTSD is a type of anxiety condition that develops after a person either directly experiences or witnesses a traumatic event such as significant injury, combat, sexual violence, natural disaster, or real or threatening death. 6 Military personnel, first responders, and police officers are at a higher risk of developing PTSD, but anybody can develop it.

Symptoms of PTSD Include:

- Detachment from others

- Irritability

- Difficulty concentrating

- Hypervigilance

- Exaggerated startle response

- Difficulty remembering the traumatic event

- Negative beliefs about oneself or the world

- Difficult sleeping

- Self-destructive behaviors

- Persistent inability to feel positive emotions such as happiness and satisfaction

- Persistent negative emotions such as fear, horror, and guilt

- Avoidance of triggers associated with the traumatic event

When exposed to triggers, intrusive symptoms such as recurring and involuntary memore, dtream, docatve responses or flashbacks, and psychological distress may occur.

Because of developmental differences, children might experience PTSD differently than adults. The DSM-5 classifies children aged 6 and younger as having PTSD with specific symptoms that are unique to the way youngsters may manipulate the disorder. Some studies have shown that instead of seeming distressed by the traumatic event or symptoms, some youngsters may look hyperactive or "over-bright."

6. Other Anxiety Disorders

There are also anxiety disorders among those listed above. Each of these anxiety disorders has a unique symptom and diagnostic profile that is outlined in the DSM-5.1.

- Specific phobia

- Anxiety disorder due to another medical condition

- Separation anxiety disorder

- Agoraphobia

- Substance/medication-induced anxiety disorder

- Selective mutism in children

Is it true that some foods aggravate anxiety while others have a calming effect?

Anxiety symptoms might make you feel ill. Coping with anxiety may be difficult and frequently necessitates a lifestyle change. There are no dietary modifications that may alleviate anxiety, but listening to what you hear may help.

Try These Steps:

1. Consume a breakfast that includes some roten: Eating protein for breakfast will help you feel satisfied for longer and keep your blood sugar stable, giving you more energy as you start your day.

2. Consume omplex arbohydrate: Carbohydrates are known to increase the quantity of serotonin in your brain, which has a calming effect. Consume foods high in complex carbs, such as oatmeal, quinoa, whole-grain bread, and whole-grain cereal. Avoid foods containing mple carbohydrate, such as ugary foods and drinks.

3. Drnk lenty f Water Even slight dehydration might have an impact on your mood.

4. Limit or avoid alcohol consumption: Alcohol's first effect may be soothing. However, because alcohol is digested by your body, it might make you tense. Alcohol can also disrupt sleep.

5. Pay Attention to Food Institute: For some people, certain foods or food additives might cause unpleasant physical reactions. In some people, these physiological reactions might cause a shift in mood, including irritability or anxiety.

6. Strive for Healthy, Balanced Meals: Healthy eating is vital for overall physical and mental wellness. Eat a lot of fresh fruit and vegetables, but don't overeat. It also benefits to consume omega-3 fatty acid-rich seafood on a regular basis, such as salmon.

7. Dietary changes may make a difference in your general mood or sense of well-being, but they are not a substitute for treatment. Lifestyle modifications, such as improving sleep patterns, increasing social support, employing stress-reduction techniques, and engaging in regular exercise, may also be beneficial.

If your anxiety is severe or interfering with your daily activities or pleasure of life, you may require counseling (psychotherapy), medication, or other treatment.

Complications

If left untreated, anxiety symptoms can change and worsen over time. Because you are afraid of experiencing anxiety symptoms, you may begin to avoid events that were formerly significant or offered you joy. This can result in societal olaton. People suffering from anxiety disorder may also suffer from depression, obsessive-compulsive disorder, and digestive disorders such as irritable bowel syndrome (IBS).

Anxiety And Stress Prevention

Stress And Anxiety Triggers

If you are suffering from anxiety, avoid establishing unattainable goals for yourself, since attempting to complete everything at once might add to your stress and worry. Focus your time on the things you can change and dismiss the things you can't. Avoid using alcohol, drugs, or cigarettes as a coping mechanism since these might lead to poor mental health in the long term.

When Are Anxiety and Tremor Harmful?

It is possible for those who suffer from long-term anxiety to have health problems. Anxiety and stress can have a negative impact on their health over time, leaving people more susceptible to diseases such as heart disease, high blood pressure, diabetes, depression, and Parkinson's disease.

Anxiety and stress can also become harmful when people develop thoughts about charming themselves or others. In these instances, they should seek medical help as soon as possible. The same applies to if their thoughts are getting in the way of being able to go about their day-to-day life.

Anxiety and stress can be treated and there are many resources, strategies, and treatments available to enable people to understand and manage their anxiety and stress levels.

How Do You Instantly Calm Anxiety?

If you're driving, at work, or in another public place and you're feeling anxious, you should try to calm yourself down as soon as possible. While it is not always feasible to feel less anxious right away, there are a number of self-help techniques you may do to assist you feel calmer sooner. They are as follows:

- Taking a break from what you're doing

- Counting to ten slowly

- Taking deep breaths

- Talking to somebody: A friend, a colleague, a family member, or a therapist.

- Recognizing that you cannot control everything

- Thinking about what's triggered your anxiety

- Focusing on positive thoughts

Breathing Exercises To Relieve Anxiety

Breathing is such a natural action that we do it most of the time without even realizing it. However, at times of tre, breathing might become read and hallow, contributing to the feeling of anxiety. Learning about different types of breath and doing easy breathing exercises for anxiety will help you overcome these feelings.

The Race Poca Relationship Between Breathing And Anxiety

If you are stressed or anxious, your body will normally activate its fight-or-flight response. The bran does not distinguish between physical and emotional threat, but reacts in the same way, increasing breathing and heart rate to get blood to the muscle faster. The increased heart rate is to prepare you to confront a physical threat or to flee from it.

The increase in breathing, or hyperventilation, upsets the balance between our bodies' oxygen and carbon dioxide levels. You may feel lightheaded as this unbalance reduces blood flow to the brain, and your fingers may begin to tingle. Severe hyperventilation might also result in a lot of confusion.

The reaction might raise anxiety levels, exacerbating the situation. Learning to control your breathing with simple breathing exercises, on the other hand, can reduce stress and allow your oxygen and carbon dioxide levels to return to normal.

What Are the Different Types of Breathing?

There are two methods of breathing. There are two types of breathing: thoracic (from the chest) and diaphragmatic (from the abdomen).

1. Thoracic Breathing

When feeling anxious arrives from the chet, rapd, shallow breathng occurs. The technique of breathing might contribute to emotions of anxiousness since the intakes of air do not feel pleasant and can make you feel as if you are suffocating.

2. Diaphragmatic Breathing

The daphragm is a muscle located at the base of the lung. When you breathe diaphragmatically, the nucleus contracts and moves below, making more space for your lung to expand. The downward movement pushes on the tomacle and forces the abdominal wall out.

The Benefits Off Dia Phragmatic Breathing

Diaphragmatic breathing promotes the natural exchange of oxygen and carbon dioxide. It slows down the heart rate and may reduce blood pressure. The knock-on effect is that we feel more relaxed, and our anxiety levels fall.

A Simple Breathing Exercise To Alleviate Anxiety

- Use this easy breathing exercise to help reduce anxiety. When finishing the workout, you can stand, ttng, or lyng. However, focus on relaxing your body and ensuring there is no tension in your houlder.

- Inhale deeply through your nose and concentrate on this action inflating your abdomen. The increase in your chet should be minimal.

- Keep your jaw muscles relaxed and exhale slowly and steadily through your mouth. It is to follow your lp lightly and make a whooshing ound with your exhale.

- Repeat this breathing technique calmly and steadily for a few minutes.

- If breathing in this manner makes you feel more anxious, stop. It may take some practice to feel the benefits of this approach, so start small and build up gradually.

- Along with these breathing techniques, several natural substances can help you relax, reduce anxiety, and improve your sleeping patterns.

How to Sleep Better If You're Anxious

Getting enough shut-eye every night is critical for our physical and emotional wellness. When we sleep, our bodies conduct a range of jobs, ranging from repairing damaged cells to boosting our immune systems. Sleep is also crucial for our brain because it allows it to integrate all of the information we've absorbed during the day and consolidate it into long-term memory.

If you don't get enough sleep every night, you'll feel tired the next day, much more irritable, and likely have lower concentration levels. They may all have a huge impact on your day-to-day life and may exacerbate any anxiety you're experiencing.

How Much Sleep Do We Require?

Experts agree that getting between eight and nine hours of sleep every night is a desirable goal. Nonetheless, good ualty sleep is required to properly nourish our brains and bodies. That means doing nothing when your body can complete three to four REM sleep cycles.

How to Sleep While Anxious

If you find yourself waking up at night with a thousand thoughts racing through your mind, you might be looking for some relaxation strategies. Fortunately, there are various things you can do to assist encourage sleep when you're feeling anxious:

1. Create a Relaxing Bedtime Routine

You must wind down appropriately and avoid potentially dangerous circumstances in the few hours before going to sleep. Creating a bedtime ritual is a great way to do this, whether it's reading every night before bed, doing some gentle yoga, or taking a warm bath to soothe your muscles. To establish a regular sleep habit, try to go to bed at the same time every night.

2. Ensure that our room is cool and comfortable.

According to research, sleeping in a colder area is better for promoting sleep. That's because our bodies naturally cool down while we sleep, causing our heart rates to drop and our blood circulation to slow down. Before going to bed, turn the heating off or down, close all the curtains properly, and make sure your bed is as comfortable as possible.

3. Experiment with Medtaton or Deep Breathing Exercises.

If you've tried counting heep and come up empty-handed, try a breathing exercise instead. You may find several apps online, such as Calm, that will lead you through meditation exercises and deep breathing regimens.

How to Help Someone Who Is Anxious

If you want to help someone close to you deal with anxiety, it's natural to feel a little out of your depth at first. While pinpointing the source of someone's anxiety might help them feel better, there are a number of other things you can do to help.

How Do You Calm Someone Who Is Anxious?

If you know someone who is anxious or experiencing a panic attack, there are certain things you may do to help them feel better.

1.Ask how you can assist them.

They may already have certain choking strategies that they use, such as They would benefit from you breathing exerce or key phrae with them.

2.Encourage them to seek assistance.

Offer to make an appointment with their GP and accompany them, or assist them in finding a epeke or just exploring the ropke options open to them.

3. Be as Understanding As Possible

Stress and anxiety may be overpowering for those who suffer from them. Asking them how they are feeling and learning more about their situation, as well as conducting your own research, will help you understand what they are going through.

They should suggest Attempt a Herbal Remedy

For decades, herbal medicines have been used to aid persons who suffer from anxiety.

1. Valerian root has been employed for hundreds of years as a herbal remedy for anxiousness, anxiety, and nausea, based only on traditional use. It has the ability to relax muscles and reduce brain activity, making you feel calmer.

2. St John' Wort another millennia-old herbal remedy used only for traditional usage to treat symptoms of moderate anxiety. St John's Wort is supposed to function by shortening the time it takes the brain to use up serotonin - the body's "happy hormone."

Don't put pressure on them to do something they aren't comfortable with. This will most likely make them feel more anxious.

Even if they believe you are unable to assist them at this time, you may be able to assist them at a later date. What's more, knowing you're there to support them is a great help in and of itself.

Ask them to breathe into a paper bag - you should never encourage someone to breathe into a paper bag during a panc attack. It is not recommended, and it may not be safe.

Explanation Of Depression

What Is Depression?

Depression is a mood or mental state characterized by a sense of loss of self-worth or guilt, as well as a diminished ability to enjoy life. A person who has been depressed and has experienced a number of the following symptoms: feeling of adne, hopelene, or pessimism; diminished elf-eteem and heightened self-depreciation; a decline or loss of ability to take pleasure in routine activities; decreased energy and energy; slowness of thought or action; loss of appetite; and disturbed sleep or insomnia

What is depression, and what can I do about it?

Depreon is a mood illness that causes a continuous sense of melancholy and loss of interest. It affects how you feel, think, and behave and can lead to a variety of emotional and physical problems. It is also known as a major depression disorder or clinical depression. Depression, often known as major depression disorder, is a mood disorder that causes you to feel chronic adne or a lack of interest in life.

Most people experience adversity or depression at times. It's a typical reaction to life's difficulties. But when ntene adne includes feelings of helplessness, hopelessness, and worthlessness that last for several days and keep you from living your life, it may be other than sadness. You might have clinical depression, which is a treatable medical condition.

416

You may experience difficulties doing routine day-to-day activities, and you may feel as if life isn't worth living at times. More than just the color blue, depression is a mental illness that cannot be "snapped out of." Depression may need long-term therapy. But don't be disheartened. Most people with depression feel better with medication, psychotherapy, or both.

Depreon varies from simple sadness or grieving, which are natural emotional responses to the loss of loved people or items. Where there is clear ground for a person's unhappiness, depression is regarded to be present if the depressed mood lasts a disproportionately long time or occurs around the precipitating event. The distinction between the duration of depression, the context in which it occurs, and certain other characteristics that underpin the classification of depression into different categories. Examples of different types of depression include bipolar disorder, major depressive disorder (clinical depression), persistent depressive disorder, and emotional affective disorder.

Depression Symptoms

- According to the DSM-5, a manual used by clinicians to diagnose mental illnesses, you have depression if you experience five or more of the following symptoms for at least two weeks:

- Your mood is low for the most of the day, especially in the morning.

- You are tired or have a lack of energy practically every day.

- You feel useless or guilty almost every day.

- You get a feeling of hopele or pemtc.

- You have a difficult time focusing, recalling details, and making decisions.

- You feel restless or slowed down..

- Almost every day, you take pleasure in a variety of activities.

- You often think about death or suicide (not just a fear of death).

- You've lost or gained weight.

- ·You can't sleep, or you sleep too much almost every day.

You May Also:

- Feel shaky and restless.

- Lose enjoyment in your life.

- Eat too much or stop feeling hungry.

- Have ache, pan, headache, cramp, or digestive problems that do not go away or improve with treatment?

- Have sad, anxious, or "empty" feelings

Symptoms

Although depression can occur just once in a lifetime, most people have several bouts. During thee epochs, ymptom accur mot of the day, nearly every day, and may include:

- Feelings of melancholy, tearfulness, emptnes, or hopelessness

- Angry outburst, rrtablity, or frutration, even over small matter.

- Loss of interest or pleasure in most or all normal activities, such as ex, hobby, or sport.

- Sleep disturbances, such as insomnia or excessive sleeping.

- Tredne and lack of energy, so even minor tasks need extra effort.

- Reduced appetite and weight loss or increased need for food and weight gain

- Anxiety, agitation, or restlessness

- Sluggish thinking, speaking, or muscular movement.

- Feelings of worthlessness or guilt, focusing on past mistakes or self-blame

- trouble thinking, concentratng, makng decon, and rememberng thing. fr e uent or recurrent thought of death, suicidal thoughts, suicidal attempts, or suicidal

- Unknown physical problems, such as back discomfort for headaches.

For many people suffering from depression, symptoms are severe enough to interfere with daily activities such as work, school, social activities, or relationships. Some people may feel generally miserable or depressed without knowing why.

Types Of Depression

- There are several types of depression disorders that a doctor can diagnose, including:

- Unipolar major depolarization.

- Persistent depressive disorder, also known as dysthymia, occurs when depression lasts for at least two years.

- Disruptive mood dysregulation disorder occurs when children and teens become highly crank, furious, and frequently have intense outbursts that are more ever than a child's usual reacton.

- Premenstrual dysphoric disorder occurs when a woman experiences significant mood difficulties before to her menstruation, which is more severe than туриста prementrual yndrome (PMS)

- Subtance-indeed mood disorder (SIMD), when symptoms occur while using a drug or consuming alcohol, or after you stop.

- Depreve disorder as a result of another medical problem.

- Another drive dorder, uch a mnor depression.

Causes

I'm not sure what depression is. With many mental diseases, a variety of factors may be involved, such as: Depression is a complex disease. Nobody knows what causes it, however it can occur for a number of reasons. Some people experience depression throughout a erou medcal llne. Others may experience depression as a result of a life change, such as a move or the death of a loved one. Others, however, have a family history of depression. Those who do may suffer from sadness and feel overwhelmed by adne and lonelne for unknown reasons.

What are the main causes of depression?

Many factors can raise the likelihood of depression, including the following:

1. Abuse: Physical, sexual, or emotional abuse might make you more sensitive to depression later in life.

2. Age: The elderly are at a higher risk of depression. That can be exacerbated by other factors, such as living alone and lacking local support.

3. Medicaton: Some medications, such as otretnon (used to treat acne), the antiviral drug interferon-alpha, and corticosteroids, might increase your risk of depression.

4. Conflect: Depreon n omeon who ha bologcal vulnerablity to it may result from personal conflect or dpute with famly member or frend.

5. Death Or Loss: Though natural, sadness or grief following the death or loss of a loved

one might raise the risk of depression.

6. Gender: Women are twice as likely as males to be depressed. Nobody knows why. The hormonal changes that women experience at various stages of their lives may play a role.

7. Gene: A family history of depression may increase the risk. It is assumed that depression is a complex characteristic, which means that there are likely many separate genes that each have a little effect, rather than a single gene that contributes to depression. Depression's genetics, like other mental disorders, are not simple or easy genetic diseases like Huntington's chorea or cystic fibrosis.

8. Major Event: Even pleasant events like beginning a new job, graduating, or getting married might cause depression. So may relocating, leaving a job or coming back, being dvorced, or retiring. However, clinical depression is never just a "natural" reaction to traumatic life circumstances.

9. Other Personal Problems: Problems such as social isolation owing to other mental illnesses or being cast out of a family or social group can all contribute to the risk of developing clinical depression.

10. Subtance Mue: Nearly 30% of those with substance abuse issues also have major or clinical depression. Even if drugs or alcohol temporarily improve your mood, they will eventually worsen your depression.

Risk Factors

- Depression often begins in the adolescent, twenties, or thirties, although it can occur at any age. Women are diagnosed with depression at a higher rate than males, which may be due in part to women's proclivity to seek therapy. Factors that appear to increase the likelihood of developing or triggering depression include:

- Certain personality qualities, such as poor elf-eteem and being too reliant, elf-crtcal, or pemtc.

- A traumatic or traumatic event, such as physical or sexual abuse, the death or loss of a loved one, a difficult relationship, or financial issues.

- Blood relation with a history of depression, bipolar disorder, alcoholism, or suicide.

- Being a lesbian, homosexual, bisexual, or transgender person, or having variation in the development of genital organs that aren't male or female (nterex) in an unsupportive situation.

- History of other mental health disorders, such as anxiety disorder, eating disorder, or post-traumatic stress disorder

- Abuse of alcoholic beverages or recreational drugs

- Serious or chronic illness, such as cancer, stroke, chronic pain, or heart disease.

- Certain medications, such as certain high blood pressure medications or sleeping pills (see your doctor before discontinuing any medication).

Complications

- Depression is a serious disorder that may have a devastating impact on you and your family. If depression is not addressed, it can lead to emotional, behavioral, and physiological problems that influence every aspect of our lives. Examples of depression-related problems include:

- Obesity is excess weight, which can contribute to heart disease and diabetes.

- Pan or bodily illness

- Misuse of alcohol or drugs.

- Anxiety, panic disorder, or social phobia.

- Family conflict, relationship troubles, and work or school problems

- Sucdal feelingng, ucde efforts, or ucde

- Cutting oneself is a kind of self-mutilation.

- Premature death due to a medical condition.

Prevention

There is no sure way to avoid depression. However, these techniques may help.

Take actions to reduce stress, increase your resilience, and raise your self-esteem.

Reach out to family and friends, especially during times of crisis, to help you weather the storm.

Get therapy at the earliest sign of a problem to help prevent it from worsening.

Consider seeking long-term maintenance therapy to help prevent a return of mtm.

What Illnesses Occur With Depreon?

It is typical for people to have other medical or mental health problems in addition to depression, such as anxiety, obsessive-compulsive disorder, psychiatric illness, phobias, drug abuse disorders, and eating disorders. If you or a loved one is experiencing signs of depression or any mental illness, see your doctor. Treatment can be beneficial.

Depression Diagnosis

Your doctor will use a variety of approaches to diagnose you with depression, including:

Physical Exam: Your doctor will examine your overall health to see whether you have another condition.

For example, you may have blood testing done to check on particular hormone levels.

Pychatrc voluton: Your doctor will be interested in your mental health and will inquire about your thoughts, feelings, and behavioral patterns. You may also complete a questionnaire.

Depression Treatment

If you or someone you know is experiencing symptoms of the condition, see your doctor. They can assess you and either treat you or refer you to a mental health professional. The sort of therapy your doctor suggests will be determined by your symptoms and how severe they are. You might require one or more of the following:

1. Medication: Most people with depression benefit from antidepressant medicines in combination with treatment. There are several types of andreas. You may have to test many kinds before you locate the one that works best for you. You may require a combination of two. Alternatively, your doctor may prescribe another type of medication to help your antidepressant work better, such as a mood stabilizer, antipsychotic medication, anti-anxiety medication, or stimulant medication.

2. Psychotherapy: Talking to a mental health expert about your depression and other issues on a regular basis might help alleviate the symptom. There are several methods available, including cognitive behavioral therapy (CBT) and talk therapy.

3. Hospital or Residential Therapy: If your depression is severe enough that you are unable to care for yourself or others, you may require psychiatric treatment in a hospital or residential facility.

4. Electroconvulsive Therapy (ECT): Brain stimulation therapy sends electric currents into your brain to help your nervous system perform better. Typically, you would not use therapy unless antidepressants are not functioning or you are unable to take them

for another health reason.

5. Transcranial Magnetic Stimulation (TMS): Your doctor will usually recommend this only after antidepressants have failed. The procedure uses a coil to send magnetic pulses into your brain to stimulate nerve cells that govern your mood.

Anxiety and the Alkaline Diet

Dr. Seb has demonstrated that a more alkalized body is superior to a body that is very acidic. An асдс body is the source of mucus, making the boy susceptible to sickness through planet-baed food, which we might all benefit from in any case. Dr. Seb's recommended food lists and alkaline recipes may be found in a variety of places. This essay will explain a little more about Dr. Seb, his approach to promoting health, and demonstrate recipes using components from his nutritional guide.

What Exactly Is An Alkalne Diet?

An alkaline diet is intended to help balance the blood pH level of your body's fluids, including your blood and urine. Dr. Seb was an herbalist who created a plant-bd veron of the det) wa alkalne ah det, acd ash det, ph det, acd ash The mineral density of the food you eat influences your pH level. All living organisms and life forms on Earth rely on maintaining a proper pH level, and it is frequently stated that disease and disorder cannot take root in a body with a balanced pH.

The acd ah hypothesis contributes to the formulation of the alkaline diet. According to research published in the Journal of Bone and Mineral Research, "the acd-ah hypothe suggests that proten and grain food, with a low potaum consumption, create a det acid load, net acd excretion (NAE), increased urine calm, and release of calcium from the

The alkaline diet seeks to prevent this from happening by carefully evaluating food pH levels in order to decrease dietary acid intake.

Your pH ranges between 7.35 and 7.45 depending on the time of day, your diet, what you just ate, and when you last used the restroom. If you have electrolyte imbalances and often consume too many acdc meals, also known as acid ash foods, your body's changing pH level might result in higher "acidosis."

Best Alkaline Foods

Although you do not have to be a vegetarian to eat a high alkaline diet, the diet is mostly plant-based. Here is a list of meals to emphaze the most:

1. Promote lkalnty with fresh fruits and vegetables The majority of: Which are the

greatest options, for example, are bananas alkaline? How about broccoli? Mushrooms, ctru, date, raisins, pnach, grapefrut, tomatoes, avocado, ummer black radh, alfalfa gra, barley grass, cucumber, kale, jcama, wheatgra, broccol, and oregano.

2. RAW Foods: Try to consume a large amount of your produce raw. Uncooked fruits and vegetables are considered biogenic or "life-giving." Cooking food depletes mineral content. Increase your intake of raw meals, as well as dry juicing or lightly boiling fruits and vegetables.

3. Plant Progeny: Almonds, navy beans, lima beans, and most other beans are wonderful choices.

4. Water that is alkaline.

5. Green Drink: Well, Drinks produced from green vegetables and grae in power form are high in alkalinity-forming nutrients and chlorophyll. Chlorella is structurally similar to blood and aids in blood alkalinization. Other foods to eat on an alkaline diet include sprout, wheatgrass, kamut, fermented soy products such as natto or tempeh, and seed.

Dr. Sebi: Food Therapy

Dr. Sebi connects the dots between physical/mental disease and depression. A malnourished person, someone who is deficient in vitamins and minerals, has a brain that is breaking down at night, resulting in irregular thinking and, eventually, destructive behavior. When the body has everything it requires, it travels. Hearing the intestines by eliminating toxins is associated with brain recovery. Toxins are eliminated from an alkaline diet that is free of acid-based foods. Happiness improved as the body acceded. Instability, lunacy, discontent, and volence occur when the body is very acidic.

Nature is the Life Model. We get php hate, carbonates, oddde, and bromde from nature. These are classified as food by biochemistry. Nutritionists are unnecessary if we consume proper meals. Nutritionists do not exist in elephant, bear, or any other animal.

Foods based on starch are commonly referred to as carbonic acid. It causes a reaction that produces sulfides, which rob the body of oxygen. We must eat electrified meals in order to have an electrified body. Electric meals are available at dgeton and amlaton.

Hearing encompasses every aspect of man. Healing provides peace, and there can be no peace unless the body is well.

Health Advantages

So, why is an alkaline diet helpful for you? Because alkaline meals provide important nutrients that aid in the prevention of accelerated indications of aging and a general loss of organ and cellular function.

As explaned more below, alkaline diet benefits may include lowering the degradation of tué and bone ma, which may occur when too much acidity robs us of critical minerals.

Foods based on starch are commonly referred to as carbonic acid. It causes a reaction that produces sulfides, which rob the body of oxygen. We must eat electrified meals in order to have an electrified body. Electric meals are available at dgeton and amlaton.

Hearing encompasses every aspect of man. Healing provides peace, and there can be no peace unless the body is well.

Health Advantages

So, why is an alkaline diet helpful for you? Because alkaline meals provide important nutrients that aid in the prevention of accelerated indications of aging and a general loss of organ and cellular function.

As explaned more below, alkaline diet benefits may include lowering the degradation of tué and bone ma, which may occur when too much acidity robs us of critical minerals.

2. Lower risk of hypertension and stroke

One of the anti-aging effects of an alkaline diet is that it reduces inflammation and causes an increase in growth hormone production. It has been shown to improve cardiovascular health and provide protection against common disorders such as excessive cholesterol, hypertension (high blood pressure), renal tonus, stroke, and memory loss.

3. Decreased Chronic Pain And Inflammation

A study discovered a link between an alkaline diet and lower levels of chronic pain. Chronic acidosis has been linked to chronic back pain, headache, muscular pain, mental problems, inflammation, and joint pain.

4. Improves Vtamn Absorption and Prevents Magnesium Deficiency

An ncreae n magneum is tested for the operation of hundreds of enzyme systems and physiological processes. Many people are magneum deficient, resulting in heart failure, muscle discomfort, headaches, sleep problems, and anxiety. Available magnesium is also necessary to activate vitamin D and prevent vitamin D deficiency, which is important for general immunological and endocrine function.

5. Aids in the improvement of immune function and cancer prevention

When cells do not have enough minerals to properly dispose of waste or oxygenate the body, the entire body suffers. Mineral loss compromises vitamin absorption, while toxins and pathogens collect in the body and weaken the immune system.

Cancer preventon is thought to be alkalne hft n pH due to a alteraton in electric charges and the releae of bac component of proteins. Alkalnty can help decreae inflammation and the risk of illnesses like cancer, plu a alkalne det more benefcal for some chemotherapeutic drugs that require a higher pH to act properly.

6. Can Assist You In Maintaining A Healthy Weight

Although the diet is not only focused on fat loss, according to an alkaline diet meal plan for weight loss will undoubtedly help protect against obesity. Reduced consumption of acd-forming meals and increased consumption of alkaline-forming foods may make it simpler to lose weight because of the diet's ability to reduce leptin levels and inflammation. This has an effect on both your appetite and fat-burning ability.

Because alkaline-forming foods are anti-inflammatory, having an alkaline diet allows your body to achieve normal leptn levels and feel satisfied with eating the quantity of calories you require. If losing weight is one of your key goals, one of the greatest approaches to consider is a keto alkaline diet, which is low in carbs and rich in healthy fats.

Keeping Our Bodies Alkaline

One of the foundations of Dr. Sebi's methodology is the distinction between alkaline and acidic meals, and the effects that each has on your body. When we look at our bodies, several factors such as hydration, temperature, nutrition availability, and pH cause cells and tissues to work.

The ph stands for "potential of hydrogen" and is a measurement of hydrogen ions in a certain solution - the more on, the more acidic the oluton, and vice versa. Our bodies are designed to operate within a very narrow pH range, which is approximately 7.365, which is somewhat alkaline. The pH scale has a range of 0 to 14. A pH more than 7 is alkalizing, a pH less than 7 is acidic, and a pH of 7 is considered neutral. When we consume an excessive amount of ad-forming meals, our kidneys are unable to keep up with the acid waste and begin to accumulate it in our urine. This is extremely damaging and hinders the body's ability to heal or detoxify, causing a person to be more susceptible to disease and illness. The most common symptoms that your body needs to detoxify from acid are:

426

- Brittle hair and nails

- Low energy

- Fatigue and chronic fatigue

- Digestive issues

- Low immunity

- Acne

- Infections and allergies

- Heavy breathing

- Gaining weight

Alkaline Diet Anxiety

The alkaline acid diet refers to eating according to the pH of food after digestion and our blood pH. According to the diet, food may be classified as alkaline-forming or acid-forming, with the former leaving an alkaline trace in the body after digestion and the latter leaving an acidic or alkaline trace. Because our blood is naturally somewhat alkaline, the diet recommends consuming mostly alkaline foods and avoiding acid-forming foods. According to supporters of the diet, eating this way decreases acidity in the body and promotes excellent health.

There are several benefits to the alkaline diet, which vary from controlling digestion and improving energy levels to providing antioxidant protection and lowering cancer and cardiovascular disease risks.

However, only a few of them are true benefits of the alkaline diet. The more specific claims have yet to be demonstrated to be a direct outcome of consuming mostly alkaline foods. The alkaline diet, like any other dietary regimen, has advantages.

Alkaline Acid Diet Disadvantages

The reason why there are negative effects to the alkaline diet is because everyone is different and may react differently to different types of meals. Even the healthiest food might be good for some of us but detrimental for others for a variety of reasons. For example, some people may benefit less from having more high-fiber foods in their diet, and most alkaline foods are also rich in bber. Other people may benefit from reducing their intake of animal products, as suggested by the alkaline diet, because they may require more B vitamins, and meat contains the highest concentration of B vitamins.

Although not harmful, some dietary modifications, such as eating more fruits and vegetables and eating less meat and dairy (the 80-20 or 75-25 ratio), might have a negative influence on one's health and can worsen certain illnesses. Is it true that the alkaline diet is harmful to certain people? Read on to learn about the 9 potential negative effects of the alkaline diet and why they occur.

What Are The Side Effects?

1. Diarrhea: The bulk of alkaline-forming foods are fruits and vegetables, which are also good providers of dietary fiber. Dietary fiber is good for digestive health because it improves intestinal transit time, encouraging efficient, regular, and frequent bowel movement. However, too much of it might result in muhy stools, which can cause diarrhea. And, because the diet recommends a high consumption of fruit, vegetables, and nuts, it can add up to a lot of dietary fiber. Easing into the diet, especially if you are a meat, rce, and cheee eater, and carefully selecting your meals to adjut your fiber intake to your body's r e urement, can help minimize the risks for diarrhea.

2. Gatrt: In addition, most alkaline foods are a good source of dietary fiber. And, while this may be beneficial for anybody wanting to cure constipation, prevent and manage hemorrhoids, and avoid the feeling of being poorly due to constipation, it may be troublesome for those of you who have gatrt. Despite its many benefits, dietary fiber can have an unpleasant effect on the stomach when ingested in large quantities, especially if you have gastritis and the stomach lining is already inflamed.

Most gastritis dietary guidelines advise us to consume more meat, such as chicken and some fish (light protein), but also white rice and refined grains, and to avoid fruits and fruit juice, high-fiber vegetables (fatty food and dairy) for a while.

Because too much fiber does not allow the stomach lining to repair, it continues to irritate it and worsen the condition. Because the alkalne diet recommends increasing your intake of fruits and vegetables by 75% or 80%, gastritis sufferers may not benefit from it at all, perhaps aggravating their condition.

3. Acne Reflux As someone who suffers from acid reflux, I can honestly tell that I have to watch what I eat very carefully. And if I ate according to the alkaline diet, I couldn't keep up with the letter. For example, several foods that are healthy according to both the alkaline diet and traditional nutritional standards are a no-no for acid reflux.

Horseradish is a high-alkalinity food, however it is also bad for acid reflux due to its phosphone content. And so is gnger, despite being really healthy. Tru fruits, such as tangerne, grapefruit, lime, or lemon, are alkaline and can help with acid reflux and gastritis. Garlc, onon, chives, bell pepper, cabbage, cauliflower, and Brussels sprouts are further examples of alkaline foods that are not very good for gastroesophageal reflux or gastritis.

4. Irritable Bowel Symptoms: Irritable bowel yndrome is a chronic, long-term disorder of the digestive tract that causes symptoms such as bloating, flatulence, diarrhea, constipation, stomach pain in the form of cramp, even anxiety and depression (most likely caused by a problem absorbing nutrients from food).

Symptoms may come and go, vary in severity, and be brought on by various factors. Certain foods are especially detrimental to irritable bowel syndrome.

In addition to the obvious (carbonated drinks, processed meals, fred and fatty foods), some other nutritious foods such as br col, cabbage, caulflower, Brussels sprout, bean, peas, horseradish, ginger, and other pce and a range of fruit The items listed as examples are also alkalne (een the alkalne acid charts), which would imply that the diet is not necessarily good for someone with irritable bowel syndrome.

5. Hunger: You will feel hungry sooner if you follow a largely vegetarian diet, which is what the alkaline diet is. The majority of alkaline foods are fruits and vegetables, which are also low in calories. Because it is calories that provide us energy, we are more likely to burn through what we eat faster and feel hungry sooner. This might be difficult since we would have to eat more frequently and possibly more than we are accustomed to, forcing us to better plan our meals. But, while it may be inconvenient for those of you with busy schedules, it may be beneficial in the long run since the diet drives you to eat healthier, more nutritious foods.

6. Bran Fog: Brain fog is associated with forgetfulness, foggy thinking, trouble comprehending and processing information, difficulty focusing, confusion, and the inability to think clearly. Nutritional deficits are one of the probable reasons for the condition. To operate properly, our brain needs lipids and B vitamins first and foremost. Both of these nutrients are available in large amounts in meat, dairy, and grains, and some people may require more of them than others (as previously said, we are all unique). However, an alkaline diet, which is largely vegetarian, reduces the intake of animal products and grains significantly, thus some people may have cloudy thinking or brain fog as a result.

7. Mood Shifts: Not obtaining all of the nutrients we require in the levels we require can have a negative influence on many elements of our health. Meat, dairy, and all grains,

for example, include vital nutrients such as amino acid and B vitamins, which are required for optimal brain function. Such nutrients are responsible for the synthesis of neurotransmitters and hormones that influence thinking, hunger, sleep, and even mood. It is possible that a diet based on animal products could result in some people not achieving their required consumption of certain nutrients, such as B vitamins, which could indirectly contribute to a negative mood, especially because a good mood is an indication of good health.

8. Risk For Anxiety and Depression: Certain nutrients are extremely important for mental health, and being lacking in them can contribute to anxiety and depression. For example, a low dpoton and a proclivity for worry and depression might be the result of an inadequate intake of B vitamins. Because the alkaline diet significantly reduces your consumption of animal products, which are our primary source of vitamin B, which is crucial for brain and nervous system function, it might lead to or aggravate anxiety and even depression symptoms.

Furthermore, a high fiber intake might compensate for nutritional deficits by lowering magnesium absorption, hence increasing depression and anxiety risk. Some plant-based foods include anti-nutrients such as phosphoric acid, which further reduces mineral absorption. Phytc acd binds to ron, znc, and calcium in particular.

9. Getting More etcde: Because the alkalne diet is predominantly vegetarian, we eat more fruits and vegetables. And because different parts of the world have different rules regarding the amount and kind of pesticides used on certain crops, there is always the possibility of ingesting more pesticides than is safe.

In realty, testing all the food reachng our dner cable and there have been report of meals contantng five or even twenty times more petcde than normal

Ways to Increase Your Body's Alkalinity

As you can see, there might be a lot of negative con e uence if your body is too асмс. An alkalne body is difficult to maintain, but it is worthwhile. If you want to balance it by becoming more alkaline, here are 15 tips on how to make your body more alkaline.

1. Check your Ph levels on a regular basis.

They provide a quick and accurate readout of your body's acidity and alkalinity levels. The result of theSE tet trip will help gude you in king your pH levels balance to your body can effectively digest important nutrients. These strips provide a practical way to test your pH level in the quiet of your own home. To test your pH, you can use either alva or urine.

The results display 15 seconds after the test is performed, and the strips include an easy-to-read chart to show you what range you are in.

2. Begin the day with a tall glass of water with a hint of lemon.

Lemon may appear to be overly acidic, yet it has a reviving effect since it helps to improve your metabolism. Clean water and a piece of freshly squeezed lemon are two of the most popular energy boosters of all time. Water with lemon offers the body pure energy through hydraton and oxygenation, providing amazing vitality and mental clarity. Fresh lemon, when added to water, helps oxygenate the body and enhances enzyme function. The fruit is known to boost the liver's natural enzymes and aid the liver in the process of eliminating toxins such as a or acid.

3. Consume Darker and Green Vegetables

When we think of nutritious food, we usually think of the color green. Similarly, when we think of nature, we think of the color green. Green is a hue associated with all of the positive aspects of life, yet when it comes to choosing what to eat for lunch, we typically avoid green meals.

Unfortunately, our taste buds have been programmed to prefer artificial flavors and sweeteners. Food manufacturers have made us seek unique flavors that can only be found in a packaged product. So, how can you convince yourself to eat more dark and green vegetables? Begin by introducing yourself to different vegetables and experimenting with them in the kitchen. You probably don't know if you'll enjoy some of these foods unless you taste them.

Also, make them easily accessible. When you reach for a snack, make sure you have cut-up vegetables on hand rather than a bag of potato chips. If you get stuck, try one of the green juice superfood powders suggested here.

4. Do More Exercise

Exercise helps your body maintain and restore its neutral pH balance of urine, as well as blood and cellular fluid. Doing aerobic exercise is the best way to maintain the acid-alkaline balance in your body since it works your muscles and can help lower the accumulation of acid in your system. When it comes to exercise, be sure to undertake at least one sort of activity every day, whether it's walking, dancing, gardening, swimming, or anything else. Also, the more you exercise, the better your overall health will be.

5. Limit alcohol consumption.

Alcohol alters your pH via affecting your kidney's ability to retain ubtance, such as phosphorus in your blood. Imbalances in blood components can significantly reduce the efficacy of your body's metabolism. When you consume a mild type of alcohol, such as beer, you are drinking a significant amount of water while also reading your kidney's capacity to eliminate that water.

This causes a fluid overload and a change in phosphate levels, which decreases the acdty of your blood, causing your pH level to increase. A single drink of alcohol might begin to alter your normal kidney function. If your liver has already been damaged by previous alcohol consumption, alcohol's effect on your kidneys will only worsen.

6. Add a teaspoon of natural baking soda to the water and drink it first thing in the morning.

Sure, it doesn't taste great, but it's a rapid method to alkalize your body. It is a simple procedure that produces immediate results. To do this, combine a teaspoon of natural baking soda in a cup of water and drink it as soon as you wake up. Among other health benefits, ingesting baking soda diluted in water helps to regulate the body's pH and promote general well-being while improving energy.

7. Reduce the consumption of acidic foods.

Limiting your consumption of acidic foods will help you maintain your pH level, prevent bone density, avoid kidney stones, and reduce the symptom of acid reflux. Foods that aid in the formation of the body should be consumed in a controlled manner. Some of these items are processed cakes and bread, cereals, eggs, peanuts, walnuts, pata, rice, oats, and cold cuts. When it comes to beverage, restrict your consumption of alcohol, milk, caffeinated drink, and beverages containing artificial weetener.

8 drink more lkalne water

You've probably heard some of the health claims made about alkaline water. While some claim that it can help slow the aging process, prevent cardiovascular disease, and regulate your body's pH level, what exactly is the hype around alkaline water?

Alkalne water has a higher pH level than regular drinking water. Because of this, alkaline water might help to neutralize the acid in your body. While regular drinking water has a neutral pH of 7, alkaline water has a pH of 8 or 9. If you can't get alkaline water, you can buy an alkaline water purifier like this one.

9. Take Multivitamin to supplement your diet.

Many of the vitamins included in a multivitamin will help you alkalize your body. Vitamins A and C, for example, boost the immune system and build the body's cells while also making the body more alkaline. Vitamin D also assists the body in maintaining an alkaline state, as well as improving calcium absorption and assisting the body in maintaining optimum mineral levels. While you may not get enough of these key vitamins and minerals in your diet, taking a multivitamin every day can help your body maintain a healthy pH level.

10. Go On A Brisk Walk.

Exercise helps you move any accumulated waste products in your body so you can remove them more effectively. Every day, go for a brk walk or incorporate another kind of cardo into your day in some way. Begin a walking regimen with a companion, and stay with it. You may even use one of these pedometers to track your steps while walking.

11. Consume Raw, Unsalted lmond

Snack on raw, unsalted almonds throughout the day to help your body combat acidity. Almonds are high in natural alkalinity minerals like calm and magnums, which help balance your body's acidity while also controlling your blood pressure.If you need to grab for some chp or cake, choose raw, unaltered almonds instead. They will keep you fuller for longer and have a better effect on the pH of your blood.

12. Reduce Your Consumption Of Sugar

Foods high in sugar, such as soda, candy, and cake, are the most acidic items you can put into your body. Sugar may be found in plan ight as well as being hdden in common food. Sugar is abundant in foods such as ketchup, yogurt, and even pasta sauce.

Sugar comes in a variety of forms, including high fructose corn yrup, artificial ugar, corn yrup solids, fructoe, ucroe, and dexter, to name a few. Sugar (in all its manifestations) is very acidic.

When you consider how common ugar is in meals (and frequently in large amounts), it is simple to see how it contributes to an unbalanced pH in the blood.

13. Reduce consumption of caffeine

Caffene is commonly found in coffee and other drinks that are intended to provide you with a pick-me-up. You could be used to reaching for a soda in the middle of the afternoon to get you through the day, or perhaps an after-dinner cup of coffee to help you finish off some work at the end of the night. However, caffeine is an acidic component that might harm your body's pH. Instead of drinking caffeinated beverages, replace them with water or tea.

14. Reduce The Amount Of Stress In Our Lives: Studies have shown that your emotional state impacts the pH level in your body. Stress affects the neural-endocrine system, resulting in greater amounts of cortisol, a tre hormone. The fact is that with any type of tre, half of the battle is realizing that the tre is working. Practicing mindfulness and recognising what is challenging you, as well as whether you are having a helpful or hindering response, is an important component of ensuring that your negative thoughts do not have a lasting effect on your body.

Developing mindfulness practices will help you become more aware of your emotions and allow them to pass without judgment. Once you're aware of your stre, take some efforts to achieve inner peace to help you cope, which will also help you keep your pH balanced and avoid harming your bones. You may also use the content platform to discover how to lessen stress and anxiety in your life.

15. Concentrate on consuming a lot of high-alkaline food.

While avoiding foods that cause your body to produce more acid, be sure to include foods that assist your body return to a more alkaline condition. Consume a diet rich in fruits, nuts, legumes, and vegetables. Consider raw Brussels sprouts, raw Swiss chard, raw mustard greens, raw eggplant, sweet potatoes, and yams. If you get tuck, Ro Brdgeford has a lot of the most alkaline food:

- Bell pepper
- Kale
- Cucumber
- Spinach
- Broccoli
- Celery
- Avocado

The Dangers of an Overly Acidic Body

Consider the consequences of having a acмc body. It can cause fatigue, headaches, chest pain, lack of appetite, increased heart rate, depression, and other symptoms. Without proper therapy, acidosis may develop into a variety of further health concerns, including kidney stones, chronic kidney disease, kidney failure, bone disease, and delayed growth. The amount of food that might cause your body to become overly acidic can certainly appear intimidating, as can the potential effects. If you're looking for a quick way to alkalize your body.

Essential Oils For Anxiety Relief

Essential Oils For Anxiety You Should Try

Eental ol has been utilized for thousands of years by those seeking anxiety treatment. They are very concentrated scent extracts. Essential oils have been around for centuries, dating back to a Biblical day when Jesus was anointed with frankincense and myrrh upon his birth. They have been used in different cultures from ancient times, including China, Egypt, India, and Southern Europe.

The beauty of essential oils is that they are natural, taken from flowers, leaves, bark, or plant roots. While it is best to use pure eental ol, which is oil that has not been diluted with chemicals or additives, they can bring much-needed comfort and healing for a variety of conditions, including a natural remedy for anxiety.

Here is our list of the top essential oils for stress and anxiety (and how to use them):

1. Essential Oil of Lavender

Lavender is possibly one of the best and most often utilized "adaptogen" nowadays, which means it can adapt to any mood. A perfect pick-me-up, the fresh and floral aroma is relaxing and calming. Lavender essential oil is wonderful for boosting mental clarity, decreasing stress, relaxing anxiety, and treating sleeplessness. The most popular of all essential oils is lavender. This miraculous cent may alleviate anxiety and treat.

When it comes to anxiety, research suggests that using essential oils topically may be one of the most effective methods to reap the full benefits. In the case of lavender essential oil, a study found that the medicinal properties of lavender entered the circulation after only five minutes of rubbing the oil on the skin.

How To Use Lavender Essential Oil For Tranquility And Anxiety:

1. Inhale Lavender I Drect For Immediate Relief Effect

Simply apply 2-3 drops of lavender oil onto your palm and take a deep breath. The smell enters the amygdala, the emotional center, and provides immediate calm. Excellent for use in the office, when traveling, or in a crowded area! If you prefer not to use the oil directly, dab 1-2 drops on a handkerchief or a cotton pad and inhale.

2. Stress Relief Headache

Rub 1-2 drops of lavender oil into your temples to relieve tension headaches. In fact, for full-body relaxation, massage 1-2 drops on the wrist or the feet.

3. tre Relief With Lavender Tea

Making a fragrant lavender herbal tea at the end of a long day may be a great way to relax. Sip and whff at the same time!

4. Lavender tre Relief ental Oil Blend: Use as a body massage oil/moisturizer. ·

- 2 drops lemon oil
- 6 drops of sage oil
- 6 tsp of carrier oi
- 3 drops lavender pill

2. Cinnamon Leaf Essential Oil

Cinnamon essential oil for treating

Cnnamon leaf ol contains anti-inflammation characteristics and works wonders for easing aching muscles and joints after a long tiring day. It can also help to minimize drowne and provide an important energy boost if you are feeling physically and mentally fatigued.

How to Use Cinnamon Leaf for Stress and Anxiety:

1. Directly inhale: Inhale the extract by rubbing it into your palm or placing 1-2 drops on your wrist or handkerchief. The spicy aroma is sure to nvgorate your ene!

2. Cinnamon Leaf ental Oil Blend for Stress Relief: Use as a full-body moisturizer and insect repellent:

- 6 drops orange essential oi
- 4 drops cinnamon leaf essential oil
- 4 tsp carrier oil

3. Cedarwood Essential Oil

Cedarwood essential oil for treamentCedarwood oil releves treatment and has a relaxing impact on the psyche. Biologically, the aroma of cedarwood promotes the release of serotonin, which is important for mood regulation. Cedarwood essential oil can also work as a natural sedative, converting serotonin to melatonin, which helps manage and regulate sleep patterns and provides a sense of peace.

How to Use Cedarwood Essential Oil for Anxiety:

1. Inhale Straight: Inhale directly from the bottle or by wiping 1-2 drops on your wrists or a handkerchief.

2. Rub directly: Rub 1-2 drops directly above your eyebrows or at the brain tem (exactly where the nick jon the heat) to relieve tension.

4. Lime Essential Oil

Ime eental ol for tre Ine eental ol, a you perhap guessed, mell just like the real thing - a freh and tart lime. It will freshen and improve the mood as well as energize without being overpowering. It may perform wonders for those suffering from the stress of weariness, bereavement, and a heavy heart, and can help to motivate a person to embrace positivism in life.

How To Use Life Oil For tre And Anxiety:

1. Make use of a Dffuer: Lme essential oil is maybe best used in a diffuser to purify the air and refresh the mood. Great for high-stress situations at work or at home.

2. Inhale in indirect: Need to get some urgent work done but just can't concentrate? Directly inhale lime oil for an instant lift.

3. Lime stress relief essential oil blend (use as a full body massage oil):

- 4 tsp carrier
- 4 drops lime essential oil
- 2 drops mandarin/orange essential oil
- 2 drops lavender essential oil

5. Grape Fruit Essential Oil

Fruit essential oil for the stress scent of fresh fruit can have amazing effect! Grapefruit, like lime, belongs to the citrus family and has an energizing, invigorating, and purifying aroma. A fantastic tre buster for fruit essential oil ecellent for mental fatgue, sadness, and stress-induced headache. An important sniff might give you the ready-to-go feeling you need to get on with your day.

How to Use Grapefruit Essential Oil for Treatment and Anxiety:

1. Use a Diffuser: Perhaps best used in a diffuser, you will be blown away by how it

makes you feel after a hard day at work.

2. Apply Topically: Add a few drops on a cotton pad along with a dab of carrier oil such as jojoba or grapeseed oil (a light oil that absorbs into the skin) and apply the blend over your wrist and neck.

3. Add to our shower: Envelope your ene by pouring a few drops to your shower and blocking the drain. To reap the maximum medical benefits, inhale deeply.

4. Grapefruit treasury essential oil combination Air Freshener:

Clean 4 oz. fine-mist spray bottle.

6 tablespoons distilled water

20 drops of Grace Fruit Essential Oil.

10 drops Print Essential Oil.

Fill the bottle with purified water and add the essential oil.

Shake, spritz, and inhale!

6. Eucalyptu Eental Oil.

Eucalyptus oil for relief, want to feel instantly refreshed? Allow the cooling impact of eucalyptus oil to work its magic. With a strong minty scent is excellent for relieving stress, boosting energy, and alleviating mental tiredness. When dealing with a cold, congestion, or the flu, Eucalyptus oil is quite beneficial. If you're feeling lethargic and intellectually exhausted, use this potent essential oil to revive and stimulate your mind and body!

How to Use Eucalyptus Essential Oil for Stress and Anxiety:

1. Include in Our Shower: Add a few drops to your shower and cover the dran. In order to reap the full medical benefit, inhale deeply. Worked really well for clearing congestion and elevating mood!

2. APPLY TOPICALLY: Rub a few drops into your temples, wrists, feet, and aching muscles and let the cooling, tingling sensation relax your muscles after a long day. To relieve a cold, massage it into your chest and back.

3. Eucalyptus stress alleviation essential oil combo Freshener.

Fill the bottle halfway with distilled water and add the essential oil. Shake and spray your pillow for a long-lasting effect, and sleep soundly all night.

7. Koe Essential Oil Rose essential oil for three tiny dab all you need to feel the powerful

effect of roe essential oil - wonderful for tmulatng the mind and creating an ene of peace, tranquility, and well-being Among all essential oils, it has the highest vibrational frequency at 320 MHz. In comparison, lavender vibrates at around 118 MHz, a healthy person vibrates at approximately 62 to 68 MHz, and so on. Roe ol is excellent for persons suffering from depression. It boosts self-esteem and encourages feelings of joy and hope.

How to use rose I for stress and anxiety:

1. Drectly inhale: Inhale immediately from the container or by rubbing 1-2 drops between your hands or on a handkerchief.

2. Directly rub: Apply 1-2 drops to your wrist and neck for a quick pick-me-up.

8. Tea TREE Essential Oil

Tea tree eental ol for tree eental ol for tree eental ol for tree eental ol for tree eental ol for tree eental ol f Tea tree oil, well known for its anti-dandruff and acne-fighting characteristics, works well in combination with other essential oils to soothe the nerves.

How To Use Tea Tree Oil To Relieve Stress And Anxiety:

1. Add the following to our hower: Infuse the ene with a few drops of tea tree essential oil in your hower. Cover the drain and inhale the goodne. Alternatively, you can add a few drops of tea tree oil and eucalyptus oil to a hot bath along with 1/4 cup Epsom salt and soak your worries away.

2. Tea tree stress relief essential oil blend Air Freshener:

- Clean 4 oz. fine-mist spray bottle
- 6 tablespoons of distilled water
- 10 drops Tea Tree Essential Oil
- 6 drops Eucalyptus Essential Oil
- 4 drops Lavender Essential Oil

Fill the bottle with purified water and add the essential oil. Shake and spray your surrounds, and let your tré melt away.

Sandalwood Essential Oil

Sandalwood essential oil for those seeking enhanced mental clarity and focus? When dealing with the demanding demands of the daily grind, having a moment of harmony and peace is crucial for your general well-being and mental health. With its beautiful woody scent, sandalwood oil has a powerful therapeutic effect on the bran' lmbc system and is an excellent emotional balancer.

How to Use andalwood Oil to Treat Stress and Anxiety:

1. Direct inhalation: Inhale drect from the battle, rubbed to the palm, or 1-2 drops on your wrt or handkerchef. Great for using before a yoga class, prayer, or meditation time to get in the mood.

2. Use Topcally: To get through a difficult day, rub a couple of drops directly on the wrist and ankle.

3. Sandalwood treasury essential oil combo (use as a whole body massage oil): 6 drops sandalwood essential oil 2 drops rosemary essential oil

4 teaspoon carrier oil

Ylang Essential Oil

Ylang essential oil for the another effective "adaptogen," lang ylang essential oil can be both stimulating and relaxing depending on how the person using it feels. It is very beneficial for dealing with anger-india tre and can provide an immediate sense of serenity and peace.

HOW TO USE YLANG YLANG L FOR TREATMENT AND ANXIETY:

1. Use Topcally: To calm agitation, rub a few drops immediately on the wrist, neck, foot, and back (trigger point).

2. Use in a diffuser: Ylang ylang essential oil works nicely in a diffuser and is thought to have aphrodisiac effects - great for elevating the mood!

3. Ylang-ylang treasury essential oil diffuser blend:

2 drops lavender essential oil 1 drop clary sage essential oil 1 drop ylang ylang essential oil To use as a massage blend, add 4 tsp carrier oil (such as coconut, grapeseed, or olive oil) to the above formula.

11. Eental Clary Sage Oil

Clary sage eental ol for tre vare sage eental ol not only ha hown to potently nfluence the levels of jane (the feel Clary sage oil is a natural antidepressant and one of the greatest anxiety cures with no side effects. Excellent for boosting mood, it helps to relieve anxiety by soothing the mind while boosting self-esteem and confidence.

1. Direct inhalation: Inhale drect from the battle and place 1-2 drops on your wrists or a handkerchief.

2. Ue n A Diffuer: When you're feeling depressed, mix 6 drops of clary sage oil with 2 drops of orange oil and experience the difference.

3. Add to our list: Add a few drops of clear agave oil to your shower and ran. Inhale deeply to relieve tension and boost your mood.

12th. Jane Dental Ol Jane essential ol for the derved from the jasmine flower, current research suggests that Jasmine oil is as excellent as "valium" at calmng the nerve and overcoming tre. Traditionally, jamne ol has been used for centuries as a natural remedy for anxiety, sleeplessness, low libido, and depression, and modern research shows that our ancestors understood what they were doing.

Jasmne ol not only alleviates sadness, but it also stimulates the intellect, helps to elevate the mood, and promotes feelings of confidence and optimism.

How to Use Jasmine Oil for Treatment and Anxiety:

1. Inhale Drect: Inhale drect from the bottle by placing 1-2 drops on your wrists or a handkerchief.

2. Topically: Rub a couple of drops immediately on the wrist and ankle to relieve anxiety.

3. Jasmine stress relief essential oil diffuser blend:

- Add 4 tsp carrier
- 3 drops grapefruit essential oil
- 1 drop ylang ylang essential oil
- ·1 drop jasmine essential oil

13th. Frankincense Essential Oil

Rich in euterpene, molecular structure what can travel through the blood-brain barrel, frankncente eental ol can help relieve the negative effects of both anxiety and depression. frankncene is obtained from the ren of the Boswellia carteri/acra tree, which is known to grow in harsh, barren, and ard conditions. Frankincense is commonly associated with many different faiths and is said to increase intuition and spirituality.

How To Use Frank Cene L For tree And Anxiety:

1. Use A Dffuer: After a long, exhausting day, diffuse a few drops of frankncene ol in the

air to experience full relaxation.

2. To our hower: Pour a few drops into a heated hower and cover the dran. Inhale deeply and let your thoughts drift away.

3. Frankincense treasury essential oil massage blend:

- 2 drops Lemon
- 4 drops Jasmine
- 4 tsp carrier oil
- 4 drops Frankincense

14. Eental Lemongras Ol Lemongra eental ol for tre aromatc, calming scent of lemongra watng through the ar can transfer you to another world. That being said, aromatherapy is one of the best methods to use lavender oil to ease anxiety, anger, nausea, and stress. Breathing in the fresh scent of lemongrass oil helps relieve anxiety symptoms and promote relaxation.

HOW TO USE Lemongra OIL FOR TREES AND ANXIETY:

1. Diffuser Application: Put a few drops of lemongra essential oil in the air and let the mild, fragrant scent revitalize you.

2. Inhale Direct: Inhale direct y from the battle of rub 1-2 drops in your palms and cup to your face. You can also put 1-2 drops on your wrists or a handkerchief or your pillow before you sleep.

3. Lemongrass stress relief essential oil massage blend:

- 4 tsp carrier oil
- 2 drops Lavender oil
- 8 drops Lemongrass oil

Peppermint is a must-have. Old Peppe Rmnt esental ol for the tre you may think peppermnt oil an excellent breath freshener, but it certanly does a lot more! Peppermint oil contains menthol, a natural anesthetic that provides an amazing, cooling sensation (think of the pleasant taste of peppermint gum).

It is important to note that peppermint oil is far more potent than other essential oils and should be used in conjunction with a carrier oil such as fractionated coconut oil, jojoba oil, or sweet almond oil. With its energizing smell, peppermnt ol keeps you alert, helps you concentrate, and alleviates feelings of mental tiredness and restlessness.

How to Use Peppermint Essential Oil for Stress and Anxiety:

1. Use n A Diffuer: Diffue a few drops of peppermint essential oil in the air to improve focus and boost mental concentration.

2. Inhale Drect: Are you feeling drowsy at work? Inhale directly from the bottle or dab a drop under your nose for a quick pick-me-up.

3. To relieve mental and physical weariness, massage a few drops to the back of the neck and shoulders for a cool, refreshing, and invigorating sensation.

Side Effects And Warnings

Essential oils are natural yet potent. Some people may develop an allergic response to any ol, so it's always better to start small by doing a small patch test on your arm or leg (never your face or neck) to ensure you don't have an adverse reaction. If you are pregnant or breastfeeding, or if you are on any medication, please consult your doctor before using this product.

What Should You Look For When Purchasing Essential Oils?

When purchasing essential oil, ensure that the bottle contains 100% pure essential oil and has the proper name of the product listed on the label. Example of lavender: (Lavandula Hybrida Medicus). When you see the word 'fragrance,' it almost invariably means there are other ingredients.

It is usually preferable to get essential oils from an organic source that are branded "Therapeutc grade," which means they are devoid of toxins and chemicals and are unfiltered and undiluted.

Dr. Sebi's Solution

Managing Anxiety in Difficult Times

Are you concerned about your mental health during these trying times? Continue reading to learn how to manage stress and anxiety.

We are at a period of great uncertainty, and many people are experiencing fear and worry as a result of olation and the potential of infection. Anxiety and stress may activate your body's flight-or-fight reaction, releasing a torrent of chemicals and hormones, such as adrenaline, into your system. While anxiety is a typical reaction to some occurrences, if you feel anxious and worried often or for an extended period of time, your body never receives the signal to return to normal functioning. This can weaken your immune system, making you more susceptible to viral infections and frequent Ilnee.

Your Immune Ability

Official figures show that those with a stronger immune system and better health are considerably more resistant to vru and t symptoms. Your immune system provides you with optimized defense, combat, and repair technology.

Every point of your blood contains 3 billion specialized phagocytes that consume viruses and germs. You're also fortunate to have specialized cells that recognise and pursue foreign invaders. Mother Nature created our immune system to keep us safe; without many safety mechanisms, we would not have lived as a species. There is a delicate balance between awareness and trust, knowing that when you support your body, it is well equipped to deal with the virus and much more. While we negotiate this challenging moment, certain more difficulties may occur that jeopardize your mental health:

Fear and worry for your health and the health of a loved one.

Change your sleeping or eating habits.

Difficulties leeping or focusing.

Worrying about a chemical health problem.

Increased usage of alcohol, marijuana, or another substance

Handle Stress And Anxiety While Self-Isolating

Maintaining your mental health and peace of mind is equally important at this time. Remove yourself from the new. Even while it is critical to be informed throughout the crisis, limit the amount of time you spend reading the news or watching social media. Only get your facts from credible sources.

1. Feed Your Body Right: It's tempting to give up and just gorge on junk food when you're in quarantine. However, it is now more necessary than ever to give your body nourishing, alkaline-electronic food.

2. Move our Body: Moving for at least 30 minutes is a fantastic method to maintain your health and cope with stress and anxiety. If you can, walk around the block, discover online yoga courses, dance about in your living room, or simply do some basic stretches before bed.

3. Make Time To Relax: Try to do something else you like. Now is the ideal moment to

read that book you've always wanted to read or binge-watch your favorite TV show. Learn a new language, or simply relax.

4. Connect with others: Tell individuals you trust about your concerns and how you're feeling.

Get Enough Sleep

Sleep is the most incredible healer. When you slow down, relax, nap, and rest, your body can focus on the task of assisting you in recovering from llne or keeping you safe. Active rest is the natural setting for many people with new lives, but now is the moment to pause and remember to let all of your energy to be focused on the body. Dr. Sebi's Nerve/Stress Relef Herbal Tea will help you enhance your mood throughout the day, and if consumed at night, it can also provide you with a mild and beep, and relaxation.

Herbal Remedies

Herbal remedies have been shown to be effective in managing symptoms and shortening the duration of the disease. The proven pottve effects of herbal therapy are controllng fever, fat clearance of chet infection, leer terod consumption, and other mtm relief. Herbal treatment may also aid in the management of tremors and anxiety.

Dr. Seb's Cold/Cough Herbal Tea helps the digestive tract recover from diarrhea by reducing mucus and phlegm. This colorful yellow flower herb and-nflammatory and revered for its ablity to reduce repratory alment.

Dr. Sebi's Banju is a tonic specifically designed for the brain and nerve system. It can help you cope with worry, stress, and depression during these tough times.

We may encourage ourselves and each other to be strong in body, mind, and spirit by working together.

Treating Anxiety

We can reduce the volume of anxious data in the network by adding underlying ue. Cannabdol (CBD) is a potent phytonutrient that can reduce our fear-induced response. Dr. Seb's Hemp-CBD product provides natural relaxation for the body and mind, reducing the excess of worry that may impair our quality of life.

The enormous increase in anxiety over the last two decades correlates with the growth in nflammatory toxn in our food, air, and water. The current increase in anxiety is linked with increased reporting of possible risks to health and financial stability. Fortunately, when the body and brain are calm and sleep is restored, nflammaton is reduced and you

445

can more clearly transmit information from the environment.

Dr. Seb's CBD helps you get out of the nflammatory cycle of fear, reducing the anxety that tell your body that omether Your anxiety needed to be rejected; luckily, Mother Nature gave healing Hemp so that we could change the deal. Find peace with CBD and change your perspective.

Stress is your body's natural reaction to challenge. In the short run, tre may be a good force, such as assisting you to reach a personal or work deadline. However, tre may be hazardous to your health if used over an extended length of time. In this article, we'll go through the most prevalent indications of stress and provide you tips on how to stress less.

We have been accustomed to the sense of stre in our contemporary environment, and it must be difficult to notice it at times. Let's take a look at some common signs of depression:

- Anxiety and agitation
- Frequent sickness
- Decreased energy
- Insomnia
- Changes in libido (sexual desire) and appetite
- Depression and general unhappiness
- Chronic pain
- Loneliness and isolation
- Digestive issues

Tips For Stressing Less

1. Make A LIST: You may believe that multitasking is the most efficient method to be productive and get things done, but this approach may be making you more stressed. If you are feeling overwhelmed by the quantity of tasks you have to accomplish, try writing everything down in a list and organizing it according to importance. Then, complete each activity individually and cross them off your list as you finish them. Seeing your conversation will make you feel more satisfied with your day.

2. Don't Ignore Self-Care: It's quite easy to become engrossed in a tornado of duties and forget about self-care. Remember, your mind and body operate best when you take care

of them. So remember to remain hydrated (one gallon of pure spring water every day, according to Dr. Seb), get enough sleep (at least 8 hours per night), and follow the Nutritional Guide.

3. Fill Up on Snacks: Sometimes life gets so busy that it's difficult to find enough time to sit down and eat a complete meal. But time should not be an excuse to disregard the need of fueling your body and mind with nutritious foods. Smoothies are quick and easy to make, and snacks like the Alkaline-Electric No-Bake Help Seed Bars are packed with minerals, antioxidants, healthy fat, and natural ugar to keep you going.

4. Take Breaks: It is critical to take frequent breaks during your workday to avoid being overworked. Set an alarm for every hour to remind you to get up from your seat, move around a little, rest your eyes, and tretch. You can vary the strategy in whichever way works best for you, such as the example below:

- Divide your task into 40-minute halves.

- Take a 5-10-minute break at the end of each 40-minute period.

- After completing three activities, take a longer rest of 30-60 minutes.

5. Relax And Recuperate: At the end of the day, it's necessary to unwind and let go of any tension. Going on a walk with a friend, spending time in nature, or practicing yourself can all help you do just that. For example, the quick and simple Hydrating Relaxing Bath may help you rest after a long day while also moisturizing your skin.

Anxiety and Irritability

Verbena tea has long been thought to have a calming effect that can help relieve stress and promote sleep. Although there have been few studies on the effects of V. officinalis on humans, there is evidence that it not only reduces anxiety and nausea, but it may also prevent the occurrence of epileptic seizures. These effects are linked to an ugar molecule in vervain known as a verbenaln, which is thought to have psychoactive characteristics.

Furthermore, mice treated with the extract spent more time sleeping than mice injected with a placebo. Anxiety, as measured by movement through a maze, would also like to improve. While it is unknown if the same effect would be observed in people, V.

Sgn and Symptom You Could Be Detoxing Too Quickly

Toxins are expelled from the body faster than they can be eliminated. More erou symptoms may appear if this occurs. Your body is sending you a warning signal to slow down and change what you're doing. Make sure your health care team is aware of any unusual symptoms. These symptoms include:

- Difficulty concentrating
- Irritability
- Anxiety and panic attacks
- Depression
- Rash
- Flu-like symptoms a very rarely vomiting
- Tension
- Tremors
- Hypertension
- Heart palpitations
- Short-term memory loss
- Muscle pain and stiffness

Support Cleansing With Herbs

Herbs have been used for centuries for cleaning and regeneration. Purifying herb improves the function of the liver, kidneys, nervous system, lungs, lymphatic system, and kidneys, as well as the elimination of toxins. When undergoing a detoxification programme, it is essential to support all of your body's cleaning mechanisms. Prevent any organism's system from being overburdened with toxins and encourage it via detoxification.

Herbs Work in a Variety How to Promote Learning 1. Hepatic herbs are those that promote liver cleansing. They have a bitter flavor and improve lver function by triggering ble flow. Dandelon root (Tarax off nale), burdock root (Arctium lappa), yellow dock root (Rumex Crpu), and Oregon grape root (Mahonia aq aquifolium) are examples of hepatc herb.

2. Duretc herb stimulates urination and aids in the cleaning of the kidneys and urinary tract. Nettle (Urt ca ca), dandelon leaf, parsley (Petroelnum crpum), and marhmallow root (Althaea Offcnal) are all excellent, gentle

3. Daphoretc herb promotes perpiration and aids the body in eliminating toxins via the kin. Effective daphoretc nclude yarrow (Achillea millefolium), gnger (Zngber offcnale),

448

peppermnt, and elderflower (Sambuca canaden).

Cleaver (Galum aparne), red clover (Trifolium pratene), prikli ah (Zanthoxylum spp.), and echnacea (Echnacea pp.)

5. Laxative herbs help with bowl cleaning. Bber laxatives, such as pyllum husks, are the gentlest. The bitter herb used to improve liver function also has a modest laxative effect. Stronger laxative herbs, such as cacara agrada (Rhamnu purhana) and enna (Senna alexandrina), stimulate intestinal transit and should be used only as a last resort in instances of tuberculosis. They can form habits and cause diarrhea and cramping.

What is a detox?

Detox diets are general short-term diets designed to eliminate toxins from your body. A typical detox diet includes a period of fasting followed by a strict diet of fruit, vegetables, fruit juice, and water. Some detoxes can include herbs, tea, supplements, and colon cleanses or enemas.

This is claimed to:

- Restore your organs by fasting.

- Stimulate your liver to clear itself of toxins.

- Encourage toxin elimination through feces, urine, and water.

- Improve circulation

- Provide your body with healthy nutrients

Detox therapy are mot commonly recommended becaue of potential exponence to toxc chemcal n the envronment or your det. These include pollutants, ynthetc chemicals, heavy metals, and other harmful compounds. These det are alo clamed to help with variou health problem, such as obesity, digestive problems, autoimmune diseases, inflammation, allergies, bleeding, and cardiovascular disease.

Toxins are prevalent almost everywhere. We breathe in the air to get to the food we eat every day. It is still difficult to eliminate toxins in our environment; but, our bodies can be strengthened from inside and our immune systems can be strengthened to withstand their damaging effects. Toxin begins to build up over time and wreak havoc on your health.

Toxin build-up can dratcally mpact and low down the effcacy of varyou organ. Some of the most common symptoms of toxic overload are listed below:

- Skin issues

- Tiredness

- Difficulty in sleeping

- Lack of focus

- Front changes indigestion constipation and diarrhea

- Bloating

Though these symptoms might be the result of any underlying medical condition, it is best to give your system a full detox every now and then, clean your body from toxins, and give it a much-needed reboot. Some of the most common txn buildup n our body nclude polluted ar, food addtve, preervatve, petcde, and fertlzer found n food Tap water or unpurified water is the main source of toxins and pollutants.

Though these symptoms might be the result of any undiagnosed medical condition, it is best to give your system a full detox every now and then, clean your body from toxins, and give it a much-needed reboot. Some of the most common toxic buildup in our body nclude polluted ar, food addtve, preervatve, petcde, and fertlzer found n food tem, proceed Tap water or unpurified water is the worst source of toxins and pollutants.

Herbs For Natural Detox

This may me make pace for creatvty, reettng ntenton, or cultivating healthy habits that support the body and mIND. It is no surprise that many look forward to "cleaning" and "detoxifying" during this time of year. While "detoxing" appears to be a modern-day answer to what appears to be an increasingly taxing environment, our ancestors have long ncorporated btter, nutrtve herb and root nto ther det. Modern science has revealed that many herbs, such as dandelion, burdock, nettle, Schandra, and red clover, have a special affinity to support the natural function of our nherent detoxification system. Honoring the age-old wdom, herbalt will continue to use these herbs to support and nourish the process rather than encouraging harmful detoxification.

Our epidermis, liver, kidneys, digestive tract, and lymphatic system all play important roles in maintaining a balance of intake and outflow flow. ncredble, nature ha proved u with a natural apo the cary of plant what are un ue enough from one another to support that.

Eat A Healthful Cleansing Diet

A healthy cleansing diet provides your body with all of the nutrients it requires to function optimally while also supporting the natural cleansing and regeneration process. To help cleanse your body, focus on fresh, organic vegetables and fruits, complex carbohydrates in the form of whole grains and legumes, easily digestible proteins like fh and tofu, and beneficial fats like extra-virgin olive oil and flaxseed oil. What you don't eat is really important. And aturated, polyunaturated, alcohol, proceed foods, caffene, alcohol, and exceve amount of anmal proten organc, freh A cleansing diet is based on vegetables and fruits.

They provide an abundance of health-protective vitamins, minerals, and phytonutrients, and are rich in soluble fiber, which aids in the cleaning of the digestive tract. Aim for even ring of vegetable and tree ervng of fruit daly (ee "How much a ervng?" at right). In general, the most colorful vegetables and fruits are the most potent sources of antioxidants. Choose dark, leafy greens over pale lettuce, and purple grid over green grid.

Include sulfur-rich vegetables such as onion and garlic, which aid in the removal of heavy metals from the body, and eat a variety of vegetables from the Crucferou family (such as broccoli, cabbage, kale, collard greens, and mustard greens), which inhibit the formation of cancer-causing chemicals.

The amino acid glutathione, found in fruits and vegetables, also aids in detoxifying. Glutathione, a potent antioxidant, aids in the neutralization and breakdown of cell-damaging free radicals, allowing them to be rapidly removed. Caulflower, aparagu, broccoli, onon, tomatoe, orange, potatoe, avocado, trawberre, and watermelon are all good sources of glutathione.

Anxiety affects people differently and can be caused by a variety of factors, both past and present. Fortunately, help is available to help people understand and manage their anxiety; the biggest hurdle is recognising it in the first place. We hope that after reading this article, it has answered any questions you may have had about anxiety and that you have found it to be a useful starting point for coping with anxiety.

Anxiety may be a crippling condition that affects every aspect of your life, from how you think about yourself to your relationships to bodily changes. Know that there is anxiety treatment accessible.

Anxiety is curable, and many people may work through their anxiety symptoms with a specific treatment plan that may include medication, therapy, lifestyle changes, and healthy eating habits.

Depression might be temporary or a long-term ailment that you learn to live with.

Treatment may not often completely cure depression, but it does typically make it more bearable. If one treatment does not work, consult with your healthcare provider. They can assist you in developing a unique treatment plan that will aid you in managing your condition.

Life is full of different streor, and we all experience some form of uneasiness every day. When anxiety levels are high for an extended period of time, pepo, you may have anxiety disorder. These disorders can be painful and debilitating, but fortunately, there are several effective treatment options. In addition to therapy and medication, you may be proactive in managing your symptoms by taking good care of yourself. Maintaining a positive outlook and keeping yourself healthy will go a long way toward reducing anxiety and increasing your quality of life.

Any natural therapy that may assist calm the mind and nerves can aid in the treatment of tremors and anxiety. When it comes to essential oils, there is no set recipe, and what works for you may not work for someone else. Because we are all biologically unique, it is recommended to experiment with a variety of essential oils, pay attention to your body, and find the "personal blend" that works best for you.

These herbal remedies are now the symbol of safety in contrast to synthetic drugs, which are seen as dangerous to humans and the environment. Although herb has been valued for its medicinal, flavoring, and aromatic qualities for centuries, the ynthetc product of the modern age has surpassed it in importance. However, the band's reliance on ynthetc is waning, and people are returning to nature in the hope of finding safety and security. It's time to promote them globally.

While lavender may help with minor anxiety, it should not be used in place of professional mental health care for any type of anxiety disorder. If you are experiencing symptoms of anxiety such as constant worrying, fatigue, nausea, and rapid heartbeat, consult your primary care provider rather than self-treating your anxiety with lavender.

There is no perfect diet for everyone, even the alkaline diet. And this is not always because the diet is unhealthy, but because we are all different and may react differently to different meals, regardless of how healthy they are. This is why alkaline foods that aid promote digestion, prevent constipation, and have a probiotic function may cause diarrhea, acid reflux, woren gastritis, and irritable bowel syndrome. Learning to modify the diet to specific nutritional requirements and selecting foods that work for us is critical for avoiding side effects.

This simple meal plan focuses on the approved nutrients included in the diet's nutritional guidelines. Meal on this plan emphasizes vegetables and fruit with a small amount of the other food group. People who want to try an alkaline diet should make sure they get enough protein. It assists in maintaining and regulating a nutritional balance in the body.

A very low proten alkaline diet can help n long weight, but it may also lead to very other health issues. As a result, it is advised to have a well-balanced alkalinity and protein-rich diet.

The sample meal plan focuses on the approved nutrients listed in the diet's nutritional guidelines. Meals on the plan emphasize vegetables and fruits with a little amount of the other food group. A diet rich in variety is the healthiest option. People should aim for a diet that includes a variety of different proteins, grains, fruits, vegetables, vitamins, and minerals.

Dr. Sebi was a naturalist and herbalist who discovered the key to unlocking a healthy body. The issue is that the way we live and eat causes an excess of mucu to build up in the body. It will cause various ailments depending on where it grows. Dr. Seb discovered that eating natural foods that alkalize the body was all we needed to do to solve the problem. An acidic body is a breeding ground for disease and troubles, whereas an alkaline body keeps your body healthy.

Conclusion

All the above information has demonstrated how doable it is to live and lead a healthy life. Most of the time, we ignore our bodies' slight alerts about impending danger. We won't have to fully collapse if we heed this message and respond by purging and flushing our system.

As we've seen, the body is designed to detoxify itself; thus, we may assist it using these Dr. Sebi herbal suggestions. You can easily combine or add these herbs to your diet to successfully maintain your kidneys' optimal function without using an artificial or scientific method.

Although we find it difficult to follow through with such processes since we are not used to them, you should make an extra effort to get the desired results. As you know, there are costs associated with everything important, and maintaining a healthy lifestyle necessitates the discipline to follow the advice emphasized in this text. All that's left to do is put your newly acquired knowledge to use now that you've learned about these herbs.

It can be quite difficult to experience social shame and psychological stress due to repeated oral herpes symptoms. Most people with any kind of herpes may learn to live with the illness, even though some of these variables substantially influence their quality of life and sexual relationships.

Aloe vera, honey, licorice extract, manuka oil, and echinacea extract are recommended topicals since they don't require dilution with a carrier oil. Herpes usually does not cause symptoms, especially in the early stages, but if you have any, it is advisable to avoid oral, anal, or vaginal intercourse. The danger of transmission is still quite significant, although some protective barrier techniques and barriers, like condoms, tend to aid and provide protection during sex.

Herpes simplex outbreaks often begin with the initial stage being extremely painful and terrible. However, this is not always the case. Some people may have outbreaks that are so mild they scarcely perceive them. When a person has moderate genital herpes, more serious outbreaks are likely to follow in a few years, and the patient may mistake the initial one for the first.

Most people only have one HSV outbreak. However, since the virus has grown more active, some people have suffered many outbreaks. Recurrence is the term used when a person has many outbreaks. Because the body is out of balance from the infection, this is generally seen in the first year. Your body's immune system is boosted by Dr. Sebi's nutritious diet and supplement, and your body starts to build and improve its defenses against the virus by producing more antibodies.

Herpes simplex virus nearly seldom causes issues in healthy individuals. Most of those who have complications include those with terminal illnesses like cancer, AIDS, etc., as well as those who are pregnant, have just given birth, or have received an organ transplant. If you fall into one of these categories and are given a herpes diagnosis, you should immediately start changing your diet and using the drugs described in this book's introduction.

I think you've decided to stop smoking permanently at this point. You've also seen how simple it is to quit smoking by implementing an alkaline-based diet, which originates from plants and herbs. Make it a rule never to touch a cigarette for any reason, regardless of how confident you are or how long you have been smoke-free. However, if given a chance to return to the moment they became addicted, all former smokers would take it

You may still live a normal life and enjoy it to the utmost whether you are suffering from cancer, lupus, herpes, HIV, diabetes, and other diseases by using Dr. Sebi's herbal cures, as well as changing your food and living a healthy lifestyle, among other things. You may live a healthy life and live longer regardless of whether these diseases have a solution. Also, for those who are not afflicted in any way, keep safe and take the necessary precautions to stay that way.

Are you happy to have read this book? Let me know!

Leave a quick review on Amazon and share your excitement with hundreds of other enthusiastic readers!

STEP 1: Scan QR Code:

STEP 2: *Leave us an honest review, we would love it if you post a video review but just a picture of the book is fine too!*

NOTE: Don't feel obligated to do so, but we would be really pleased.